THE CLEAR
SKIN DIET

THE CLEAR SKIN DIET

The Six-Week Program for Beautiful Skin

NINA & RANDA NELSON

WITH FOREWORD BY JOHN MCDOUGALL, MD

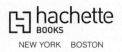

hachette
BOOKS

NEW YORK   BOSTON

Hachette Books
Hachette Book Group
1290 Avenue of the Americas, New York, NY 10104
hachettebooks.com
twitter.com/hachettebooks

First Edition: April 2018

Hachette Books is a division of Hachette Book Group, Inc. The Hachette Books name and logo are trademarks of Hachette Book Group, Inc.

The publisher is not responsible for websites (or their content) that are not owned by the publisher.

The Hachette Speakers Bureau provides a wide range of authors for speaking events. To find out more, go to www.hachettespeakersbureau.com or call (866) 376-6591.

Print book interior design by Amy Quinn.

Library of Congress Cataloging-in-Publication Data

Names: Nelson, Nina (Actor), author. | Nelson, Randa, author.

Title: The clear skin diet: the six-week program for beautiful skin / Nina & Randa Nelson; with foreword by John McDougall, MD.

Description: First edition. | New York, NY: Hachette Books, 2018. | Includes bibliographical references and index.

Identifiers: LCCN 2017052338| ISBN 9781602865655 (hardcover) | ISBN 9781602865815 (ebook) | ISBN 9781549168567 (audio download)

Subjects: LCSH: Acne—Diet therapy. | Veganism. | Skin—Health and hygiene. | BISAC: HEALTH & FITNESS / Beauty & Grooming. | BODY, MIND & SPIRIT / Healing / General. | BODY, MIND & SPIRIT / Inspiration & Personal Growth. | COOKING / Health & Healing / General. | HEALTH & FITNESS / Diets. | HEALTH & FITNESS / Nutrition. | HEALTH & FITNESS / Healthy Living. | SELF-HELP / General. | SELF-HELP / Motivational & Inspirational. | SELF-HELP / Personal Growth / Self-Esteem. | COOKING / Vegetarian & Vegan. Classification: LCC RL131 .N45 2018 | DDC 616.5/3—dc23

LC record available at https://lccn.loc.gov/2017052338

ISBNs: 978-1-60286-565-5 (hardcover), 978-1-60286-581-5 (e-book)

Printed in the United States of America

LSC-C

10 9 8 7 6 5 4 3 2 1

For our parents, Jeff and Sabrina,
whose love and support have made this book possible;
for our family's guardian angels,
John and Mary McDougall;
and for our plant-strong head coach,
Rip Esselstyn.

Special Note to Reader

If you are experiencing suicidal thoughts because of your acne, you need to seek professional help right away. We know you are really hurting, and you should talk to someone to help you get better. And you *can* get better, trust us on this.

This book is not intended as a substitute for the medical advice of physicians. The reader should regularly consult a physician in all matters relating to his or her health, and particularly with respect to any symptoms that may require diagnosis or medical attention.

Dear Reader

We are so happy you decided to check out our book!

If you're one of those people who wants to skip ahead to see just how well this diet heals acne, then turn to the center of this book and look at the full-color before and after photos. We think you'll be inspired when you meet people who have embraced the Clear Skin Diet and finally were able to get control of their skin.

Following this diet and healing our acne allowed us to continue our careers as commercial actors, YouTubers, and social media personalities. Our personal lives improved as our confidence was restored. The diet and lifestyle changes detailed in this book cleared our faces and have kept them clear for over three years—and brightened our outlook on life.

When you follow the Clear Skin Diet, you will:

- Halt new acne breakouts and start to heal your skin
- Enjoy having a sense of personal power when you gain control of your skin
- Improve your self-confidence and self-esteem
- Lose weight (unless you don't wish to)
- Improve your cardiovascular health
- Have fun learning how to make smart and delicious food choices
- Feel fantastic

The Clear Skin Diet is easy to learn and implement. You feast on the healthiest foods nature has to offer—fruits, vegetables, whole grains, and legumes—while you heal your skin. The foods we recommend don't just decrease inflammation, they are also incredibly delicious. To make your transition as easy as possible, we have included many easy recipes that will leave you not just smiling but also healthy and satisfied. Beyond the food, we've shared all our tips to develop a skin-positive face care routine and a clear skin environment.

We created the Clear Skin Diet for the many people on our various social media platforms who witnessed our transformation and who wanted to be acne-free too. For this book, we consulted several well-respected medical and dietary experts to ensure that this program is both nutritionally and medically sound. We've worked to keep the cost of food affordable and familiar, and to minimize meal prep time—while still providing delicious results. Our top goal was to create a routine that is attainable for each and every person battling acne—whether they are thirteen or forty-three.

Is the Clear Skin Diet difficult? Well, when you are regularly bombarded with advertising for junky food, or pressured by skeptical peers or family who insist that "one little bite of this or that won't hurt," it may not *always* be easy. But rest assured, you are going to be OK, and you'll actually enjoy the food. Most of all, you're going to love your new and improved skin. And who cares what other people think about how you eat? It's cool to be different.

We also want to invite you to visit us online at ClearSkinDiet.com. There you will discover additional inspiring stories and photos, special video content, and a skin-care ingredients checker. Perhaps most importantly, you can interact with many other people who are successfully doing the program!

So jump in with both feet and make a commitment to yourself. You're on your way to freeing yourself from acne. And this kind of freedom is one you will definitely enjoy!

Nina & Randa

CONTENTS

Foreword

I am excited and honored to have been asked to write the foreword for *The Clear Skin Diet*. Excited because I believe this book has the potential to end the acne epidemic as we know it; honored, because I have known Nina and Randa Nelson since they were very young children, and understand how passionate they are about assisting those who are suffering unnecessarily with this physically and psychologically painful disease.

I've had the opportunity over the last two decades to watch Nina and Randa grow from highly energetic, curious kids to the intelligent and influential young women they are today. Their personal transformation has already inspired thousands of people on social media, and now they are on the brink of helping millions of people around the world heal their skin and recover their self-esteem.

As someone who has been practicing medicine for over thirty-three years, I have personally witnessed the tragic health consequences of the typical western diet: diabetes, heart disease, hypertension, cancer—and acne. These are all diseases which negatively impact the quality of a person's life, not to mention their mortality. I have unfortunately had to do my share of prescribing the usual pharmacological suspects. But pills don't really cure, they just mask symptoms. What I discovered during my years of practice is that there is only one thing which consistently heals and cures my patients: changing their diets.

And this is where the miracle of the Clear Skin Diet begins, with food.

People suffering with acne can rejoice that they are holding the cure to their problem in their hands, right now. This book can teach you how to regain your health, and take control of your skin. It's incredibly empowering to think how easy it is to heal your skin, just by eating the wholesome, delicious foods your body is built to thrive on. Removing inferior food from our lives and replacing them with health-promoting food allows your skin to heal. No expensive pills, potions, lotions, or other treatments required.

The Clear Skin Diet isn't a fad or "designer" diet. It's a low-fat, starch-based program, like the one I've been using for over thirty years to cure my own patients. It's essentially the same diet I use to help my patients with heart disease, diabetes, obesity, etc.; it also cures acne. This is because it is a natural diet that calms inflammation, which is what acne is at its core. The research for eating the Clear Skin way is solid, peer-reviewed, and published in major journals. A wealth of research exists showing that emphasizing whole starches, and including fruits and vegetables, is the path to glowing good health.

Acne is ubiquitous in our society, but it doesn't have to be. It's only "normal" in places where the "normal diet" is consumed—a diet comprised of acne-triggering foods. The acne-promoting diet is the diet eaten by most Americans, Europeans, and Australians. It's sometimes called "the Western Diet," but it's taking hold in many new parts of the world, too. Fortunately, we know there are places in the world where no one ever gets acne. What these cultures have in common is that they consume a low-fat, starch-based diet that closely resembles the diet taught in this book.

As a doctor, it is my job to treat people for their aches and pains, injuries, illnesses, or diseases. Sometimes that means ordering tests to discover the source of the patient's problem, and then prescribing medication accordingly. But there are alternatives to curing your acne, and this book offers a "clear" choice to acne sufferers. You don't have to take medications with serious side-effects to heal your skin. If you follow the principles outlined by Nina and Randa in this book, your will be able to have the clear skin you have always dreamed of— merely by filling your plate and your body with life-affirming food.

John McDougall, MD
Santa Rosa, California

The Clear Skin Diet Team

We assembled a powerful team of experts for this book to not only make sure any advice we give is medically sound but also so that you could receive the benefit of their expertise as well. We will be sharing information we received from our esteemed panel throughout the book. This is an absolutely extraordinary group of authorities, and we're very lucky they agreed to contribute to this project. (in alphabetical order)

Neal Barnard, MD—Founder, Physicians Committee for Responsible Medicine (www.pcrm.org)

Chef AJ—Creator, the Ultimate Weight Loss Program (www.chefajwebsite.com)

Ann Esselstyn—Coauthor, *Prevent and Reverse Heart Disease Cookbook* (www.dresselstyn.com)

Caldwell Esselstyn Jr., MD—*New York Times* bestselling author, *Prevent and Reverse Heart Disease* (www.dresselstyn.com)

Jane Esselstyn, RN—Founder, Health Care Is Self Care (hcissc.com)

Rip Esselstyn—*New York Times* bestselling author, *The Engine 2 Diet* (www.Engine2.com)

Julieanna Hever, MS, RD, CPT—The Plant-Based Dietitian (www.PlantBasedDietitian.com)

Walter Jacobson, MD—Psychiatrist, bestselling author (www.WalterJacobsonMD.com)

Matt Lederman, MD—*New York Times* bestselling coauthor, *Forks Over Knives* (www.WholeFoods Diet.com)

Leila Masson, MD, MPH, FRACP, FACNEM, DTMH, IBCLC—Pediatrician (www.drleilamasson.com)

John McDougall, MD—*New York Times* bestselling coauthor, *The Starch Solution* (www.DrMcDougall.com)

Mary McDougall—Chef, *New York Times* bestselling coauthor, *The Starch Solution* (www.DrMcDougall.com)

Jeff Novick, MS, RD—Dietitian, plant-based nutrition expert (www.JeffNovick.com)

Alona Pulde, MD—*New York Times* bestselling coauthor, *Forks Over Knives* (www.WholeFoodsDiet.com)

Irminne Van Dyken MD—Surgeon who teaches a whole-food, plant-based diet (www.outofthedoldrums.com)

PART I
THE CLEAR SKIN DIET

FROM A LIFE DEVASTATED BY ACNE TO CLEAR SKIN

by Nina

"There is no single disease which causes more psychic trauma, more maladjustment between parents and children, more general insecurity and feelings of inferiority and greater sums of psychic suffering than does acne vulgaris."

—Marion Sulzberger, MD, 1948[1]

It was August 2014. Acclaimed entertainer Robin Williams had committed suicide a few days earlier. I remember walking into my parents' home office and saying to my mom, "I feel like Robin Williams."

My mom responded, "Get your swimsuit, we're going to the pool."

But I didn't want to go. I didn't want to leave the house. I didn't want to be seen in public.

Up to that point, I had been a smiley, outgoing twenty-year-old girl with a burgeoning career in the entertainment industry. Why was I so depressed that I was having suicidal thoughts and wanted to avoid contact with others?

The answer was written all over my face.

———◇———

Only a few months earlier my twin sister, Randa, and I were experiencing a dream trip in Europe. We toured England and France, stayed with family friends, and saw the sights. Much to our surprise, we were recognized by other kids. They would approach us and say, "Are you Nina and Randa? Oh, my gosh! Can I get a picture with you?"

That was unexpected, even absurd. Yes, we had a small but growing YouTube following. And yes, we had worked with Justin Bieber and were featured in one of his most popular music videos. But we didn't think of ourselves as celebrities! And yet these friendly strangers thought we were Hollywood starlets who they had to meet and get a picture with.

Being a performer seemed like a relatively ordinary occupation to us. We grew up and attended a school in the Los Angeles area—Sierra Canyon—which happens to be filled with the offspring of movie and TV stars, musicians, writers, producers, and directors. So everyone and their brother, literally, had ties to the entertainment industry.

Because we grew up as performers and had several friends whose parents are in the entertainment industry, it wasn't much of a stretch to think that a career in show business was possible. Every day after school and during summers too, Randa and I had several hours of dance and musical theater training. Our childhood normal was school and dance, school and dance, school and dance.

When we were just sixteen, a friendly conversation with a nice couple while waiting in line for a private movie screening led to our being signed by a major Hollywood talent agency. Turned out the gentleman we were chatting with was the head of the agency. After he handed us his card and told us to call him on Monday, he added, "You are going to remember this as the night you were discovered."

We signed with his agency that week and began working frequently. Overnight, we were cast in commercials, television shows, music videos, and movies and even began modeling.

We were just a couple of high school juniors who were lucky enough to be in the right place at the right time. We were booking regular gigs, having the time of our lives, and increasing our bank balances. We later applied and were accepted together at the university of our choice and made plans to attend college while pursuing our burgeoning showbiz career. The summer after graduation, however, Randa and I began to consider deferring college for a year so that we could take advantage of the professional opportunities we were being offered. We met with the head of admissions at the college, who encouraged us to "go for it." So we did.

Our career was on a roll. We starred in commercials for companies like

Nintendo, ESPN Sports as the Doublemint twins, Petco, Samsung, JC Penney, Target, Taco Bell, Google, and more.

We sweated in *17 Fit Club* workout videos as fitness trainers. We were featured in music videos with Ariana Grande; Tyler, The Creator; Miranda Cosgrove; Victoria Justice; Zendaya—even Pat Boone ("the Justin Bieber of the fifties," my grandmother said; she was thrilled). We made appearances on shows like *Modern Family, Good Luck Charlie,* and *The Neighbors.* We posed in print and catalog ads, appeared in half a dozen films, and had a fast-growing YouTube channel. We also wrote songs, gave live musical performances at various venues around Los Angeles, and produced our own music videos.

I wouldn't say that at twenty years old Randa and I were at the pinnacle of success—but we were working regularly with impressive people and having loads of fun, and our careers seemed off to a solid start.

Then the nightmare began. And our dreams started to unravel.

—◇—

Acne.

Randa and I had pretty much sailed through puberty and our teen years without suffering any real pimple problems. We were athletic and healthy, and we ate a good diet. While some of our friends were having issues with acne, we had virtually none.

But something completely unexpected happened when we turned twenty. Horrendous breakouts. The acne started gradually, and then suddenly was raging. An explosion of angry red spots materialized on our faces. Then it spread. Big, red painful zits and blackheads engulfed our cheeks, chins, and foreheads. The inflammation was so virulent, we looked like we'd contracted some contagious disease.

The acne horror began in early 2014, while our parents were away in Hawaii on a business trip. We both caught the flu and had to fend for ourselves. We were living on peanut butter and toast because we felt too sick to cook anything else. The acne got a toehold when our resistance was down. Suddenly, we were weak, helpless, and feeling increasingly hopeless. We texted photos of our faces to our mom, who told us to get to a dermatologist immediately. The abrupt acne onset looked too scary to be a normal breakout.

We rushed to Urgent Care, and the doctor prescribed antibiotics. He was disturbed by the virulence of the sudden breakout. The acne, and the flu, started to recede. Thank goodness! Maybe the acne was a temporary a side effect of the nasty flu. Unfortunately, after the initial relief, the flu went away—but the acne returned with a vengeance. Subsequent antibiotic courses were less and less effective.

Managing acne became a job. We embarked on a succession of ridiculously expensive, dermatologist-recommended oral and topical prescriptions. We tried doxycycline, clyndamycin, Epiduo, Retin-A, and Aczone, to name a few. Bear in mind that before this acne bout, we had taken antibiotics maybe once in our lives. We hadn't needed them. We slathered our faces with numerous over-the-counter creams and started getting regular facials. One facial was so aggressive I ended up with second-degree burns, which required medical treatment.

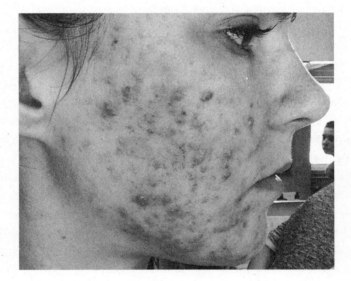

Meanwhile, our professional life was crashing. We were being sent out on the same number of auditions, but we weren't getting callbacks. If you don't get the callback, you're not getting booked.

Although we plastered on a ton of makeup to try and cover the lumps and bumps, the skin deception wasn't working. We had gotten accustomed to auditions where you had banter with the casting director, schmoozing in the audition room. Now we were being hustled in and out quickly with hardly any friendly talk. The encounters started to dent and bruise our self-esteem.

"OK, you are...?" said the impatient voice behind the audition camera.

"Nina Nelson, Daniel Hoff Agency," I said, smiling. The casting director zoomed in on my face, said nothing for a few seconds, then:

"OK, great. Thanks very much...Who's next?"

Sometimes there was dialogue for the role, and we wouldn't even get a chance to read the lines at the audition. And it wasn't just the acne preventing us from getting jobs, it was our complete lack of self-confidence. Acne had taken over our lives and was mentally exhausting. Around this time some friends at Native Foods Café asked us to do a short promo for their restaurant. I had such bad anxiety about the acne that I refused to appear on camera during the shoot. Randa did the stand-up, and I did the voiceover.

There came a point when Randa and I didn't even want to bother with auditions. Casting directors could probably sense our depression and negativity; we began to turn into young hermits, our outgoing personalities collapsing inward. We were afraid our agency was going to drop us because we couldn't get work.

We discontinued live singing and performances and only made new YouTube videos sporadically. We assumed (wrongly) that other people would be as focused on our acne as we were. We didn't even want to hang out with our friends and would turn down invites to parties. We were too self-conscious to be out in the world with our raging acne.

The worst part of all of this was that we felt totally helpless. When your skin is so completely and utterly out of control, you start to believe you've lost control of everything. We obsessed on washing our faces, trying different lotions and pills, and taking multiple trips to dermatologists and specialists who couldn't seem to do anything but offer more drugs. Truly a vicious cycle. We tried scrubs, light therapy, and high-frequency electrical currents. We changed our special satin towels, pillowcases, and sheets daily. We were frantic to discover anything that would get the acne under some semblance of control. Nothing worked. Our skin just seemed to get worse and worse, until even patches of normal skin were gone. We were at war with our skin, and we were losing. The severe acne had captured all of the territory.

Our longtime dermatologist, seemingly as confused as we were about the source of this virulent acne, finally decided to refer us to a leading acne expert at UCLA. This was basically our last hope. We waited months to get an appointment with this in-demand doctor. Our dermatologist was optimistic, reassuring us that "they have more tools in the bag at UCLA than I have here." When the appointment with the UCLA doctor finally came, however, he took one look at us and repeated what the other doctors had all agreed on: Accutane. Our hopes were dashed. He sent in his nurse to give us the "Accutane talk." We were told that the potential side effects were so severe for a baby that we'd have to go on birth control in case we got pregnant. The Pill on top of pills. As a parting gift, we were handed an Accutane information pamphlet the size of a phone book. Nothing completely terrifying about that, right?

Wrong. Accutane was not an option. We had friends and relatives who had taken it and believed it had saved their skin. We also knew others who had taken it for a short time and weren't able to tolerate it. Their skin got super dry, or their hair fell out, or they felt weird and became suicidal. One got strange rashes and very dry eyes. Another reported getting colitis and had to drop out of college to recover. Then there are the side effects they don't even know about that might show up eight or ten years after you've stopped taking the drug.

Hair loss, dry skin, depression, inflamed colon—the idea that you had to take a pill for acne that might provoke destructive side effects seemed preposterous. We became even more confused and fell deeper into despair.

One of our lowest points was in August 2014, when *American Idol* flew us to New Orleans to audition for its show. This was a major opportunity, a chance to perform in front of celebrity judges Jennifer Lopez, Keith Urban, and Harry Connick Jr. Our acne was on a rampage. We attempted to disguise our faces with heavy makeup and big floppy hats, hoping they wouldn't notice how ravaged our skin had become. The judges were all incredibly nice and supportive. Jennifer Lopez was especially kind, mentioning that she had her own twins and what a joy they were. But because our insecurity threw us so far off our game that day, the experience felt like a disaster. We wondered later why we even bothered going.

When we returned from New Orleans, we convinced ourselves that our goal to be professional entertainers had evaporated. Our careers were over before they began. We couldn't be public personalities when we didn't even want to go out in public. Randa tearfully announced she wanted to get a job at our local Whole Foods Market because she liked the people there and what the store represented. I thought maybe I could work there, too. We hoped that we wouldn't be judged too harshly because of our tortured skin.

A few days after my troubling thoughts about Robin Williams, my parents, brother, sister, and I decided to visit our grandparents. The five of us began the trek up the Interstate 5, passing through the farmland of central California to arrive eight hours later in the San Francisco Bay Area. During the daylong road trip, the conversation constantly returned to the bane of our existence, our painful acne. We cried, we whined, we expressed our despair and frustration.

At one point my dad, probably sick of our hours of carping and complaining, asked us: "What about the amount of fat in your diet? Have you thought about that? Yeah, we all eat a healthy diet," he said, "but maybe Dr. McDougall has information on acne that might be helpful? Why don't you do a search?"

Dr. John McDougall is a physician and nutrition expert in Northern California who had saved my mom's life. Literally. My mother had been diagnosed with a rare autoimmune disease in 1995 and had suffered and taken strong medications to cope with it for about a year. Then she discovered a book by Dr. McDougall and, based on Dr. McDougall's recommendations, radically changed her diet. The diet put her disease into remission, and this miracle was the reason our family had been vegan since 1996, virtually my whole life. Dr. McDougall prescribes a low-fat plant-based or vegan diet.

Back on the Interstate 5, Randa pulled up a couple of Dr. McDougall's articles on my phone. As she read aloud his observations about acne and diet and how people in parts of the world who don't eat the standard American diet don't get acne, we started to feel a glimmer of hope. Dr. McDougall described how acne was cured with a very low fat vegan diet. Nuts, nut butters, soy products, avocados, coconut—these were healthy plant foods, he said, but they could wreak havoc when hormones are running wild.

This struck a chord. I remembered when the acne had first flared, when our parents were away in Hawaii. What were Randa and I living on during that time? Peanut butter on toast—fat on bread. Bingo.

All of this sounded very logical. We decided we were going to start following Dr. McDougall's acne guidelines immediately, even while visiting our grandparents.

A new chapter in our life began with our very next meal.

—◇—

When you are afflicted with severe acne, you develop the habit of constantly examining your face. You stare in the mirror, cocking your head at different angles, searching for new red areas, new blackheads, new problems. You're instantly aware of improvement or deterioration. The obsession makes you constantly anxious. I had stared at my face so much, I knew every single spot.

So I was shocked when, after only three days of our new diet regimen, there weren't any new pimples! I recognized that I still had a lot of active zits, and my skin still looked red and inflamed, but there were no new breakouts.

To be accurate, our acne didn't just completely vanish in three days. But day by day our skin began to steadily improve. Within about two months, our acne was nearly gone! We still had some post-inflammatory hyperpigmentation and imperfections, but the active acne had finally stopped.

Take a look at our before and after photos below. The after photos were taken six weeks after the before photos. Actually, the before photos were taken almost a week *after* we changed our diet, so our actual acne was even worse than these before photos show. The after photos were snapshots we took with our phones. The lighting isn't great, but the photos reveal how dramatic the impact of the new diet had in a very short time. It was undeniable. Sometimes people have a hard time describing the intensity of their feelings regarding a significant or traumatic event. I have no problem at all describing how I felt when I started to get control over the out-of-control acne.

I felt empowered.

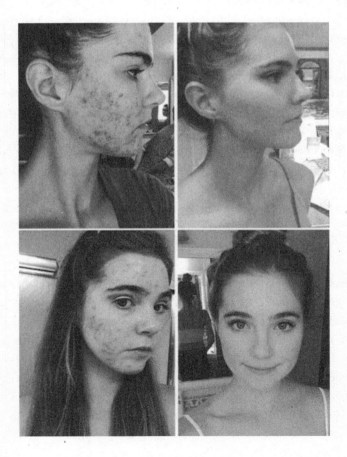

The greatest feeling in the world to someone who feels helpless is to regain control. That's how my sister and I felt, discovering that we could finally control our skin. We could regulate the acne—just by making some easy changes to our diet!

The acne nightmare was over, and our dreams could continue after all. As our skin started to recover so did our self-confidence. Two months after altering our diets, we booked a guest spot on the ABC family show *Freak Out*. We were more upbeat at auditions, and the callbacks resumed. Then we booked a string of major commercials. Humira, BMW, Big Sexy Hair, an 11.22.63 promo spot, an ESPN commercial with Jimmy Kimmel...We were back with a vengeance.

We felt blessed by our recovery, so we decided to make a video on our You-Tube channel about our acne story and how we recovered. Believe me, it's *not* easy for an actress to expose herself when not looking her best. And those before photos were truly shocking. But because our acne situation had given us such insight into the unbearable misery acne sufferers endure, we felt an obligation to open up and perhaps help a few people as we had been helped.

Much to our surprise, this acne video quickly shot to half a million views. Whoa! Thousands of kids with acne started coming out of the woodwork, kids who, like us, had tried (and failed at) everything. People with acne were intrigued by potential solutions to their biggest problem. They furiously posted questions on our channel: "How exactly did you do it? What exactly do you eat? Show us what you eat in a day. Show us what you eat every day for a week. My mom watched your video and she wants to try it too. Do you have any advice for parents? Will I get enough [fill in the blank with any number of nutrients] on this diet?"

Randa and I felt honored to be given an opportunity to help so many. We most definitely related to their desperation. "Please help me, I'll do anything to get rid of this acne!" We obliged. We dedicated a big chunk of our new videos to acne—to the tips and tricks we had discovered through research, trial, and error. And day after day we gave our recipes and advice: suggestions for breakfast and lunch for high-schoolers and college kids and health information that answered parents' questions.

Our subscribership went from around 7,000 to more than 600,000, with over 70 million views of our videos. After a while, we observed an exciting trend. A large number of people were posting that they had taken our advice—and cured their acne! They wrote on our various social media platforms or e-mailed us that they had followed our program and their acne had disappeared, just like ours. A thirteen-year-old from New Jersey, who had discovered us on

YouTube by searching "how to get rid of acne," said she binge-watched every one of our acne videos with her mom. She tried our diet and had improvement within a week, with her acne almost completely disappearing within six weeks. A nineteen-year-old girl from Kentucky said she got rid of horrible cystic acne by following our diet and was "beyond happy." A seventeen-year-old girl from New York said our diet had changed her life: within two months not only had her skin begun to clear but she had also lost sixteen pounds.

Getting messages like this made us feel almost—and this might sound a little weird—grateful for having had acne. Grateful that we could have the opportunity to be of service to people who were suffering like we had. We felt obligated to help them put their acne into the past tense.

Celebrities on YouTube began following us on social media and adopting our anti-acne diet. As word spread about our success, a major media outlet did a feature story about our triumph over acne titled "Identical twins who suffered from horrific cystic acne reveal how they cleared their skin and banished blemishes in THREE DAYS with a vegan no-fat, no-oil diet." The article explained how we stopped having new breakouts after only three days and showed several dramatic photos of our skin before and after the diet.

This piece stirred up a hurricane of attention. Within days similar articles with those memorable acne photos appeared on media outlets around the world. They were in Spanish, Italian, Russian, Hebrew, French, German, Portuguese, and Japanese. Our acne story went around the globe and back!

Soon after, TV producers from talk shows like *Dr. Oz* and *Inside Edition* invited us to reveal how we cured our acne. This flurry of attention made us realize our story was impacting more people than we had realized. We started assembling a short acne e-book to show people how to follow our anti-acne program. When we understood that a traditional published book had the potential to reach an even larger audience, we decided to go that route. Getting the message out to a broader audience meant reaching and helping more people who were suffering as we had.

—◇—

The agony of millions of children, teens, and adults generates billions of dollars for acne-related businesses. Acne is big money. Over three billion dollars is spent treating acne every year.[2] It's an epidemic for young people and adults alike. The cure that we discovered turns out to be inexpensive. It's easy, cheap, and as near as your local supermarket. And you don't have to pay for a doctor's visit or overpriced prescription drugs (which could fail you anyway). The knowledge we stumbled upon is simply this: adopt a satisfying, very low fat plant-based diet, develop a simple, clean skin care regimen, stop worrying about your face, and start living your life again!

—◇—

DIET STOPS ACNE: ASHLEY BROWN, AGE 20

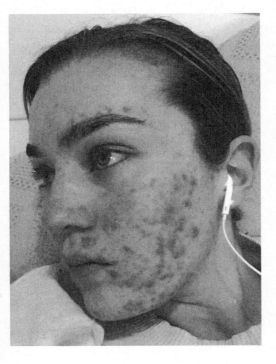

Ashley wanted to lose weight and tried a low-carb diet. She ate eggs, gallons of dairy products, and salads doused in oil. She did lose weight, and her self-confidence improved. Unfortunately, she soon discovered that her skin hated her new diet. Her face was breaking out painfully.

Ashley's stress about her acne made her become severely depressed. She decided to take a medical leave of absence from school. Ashley said: "I was so upset. My skin was horrible, and I had just left college due to depression. I felt like I had messed everything up. I had seen information on YouTube from Nina and Randa about using diet to cure acne. I read up on Dr. McDougall and decided to try this diet approach myself and to be super strict."

Ashley tried Accutane twice before, and it hadn't worked for her either time. Even if it had worked she didn't believe it would address the underlying cause of the acne.

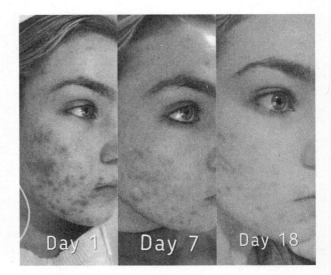

Day 1   Day 7   Day 18

Ashley followed the Clear Skin Diet principles, and in addition, she cut out gluten and processed sugar and kept fruit to a minimum. She says: "I fell in love with vegetables. I don't know how many bags of Costco frozen veggie mix I have gone through in a month. I started exercising semiregularly, mostly just for enjoyment, very light cardio." Ashley took a weekly photo tracking her progress.

Ashley's acne cleared quickly. In less than a month, she had no cystic acne. As her skin improved, she also lost eight pounds "almost effortlessly." Some months later, Ashley experimented by adding some overt fats back into her diet, including nuts, nut butters, avocado, even some oil. And she had no recurrence of acne. Some people clear their acne and then try adding back more fats—and they start breaking out again. So everyone's sensitivities are a little different. Ashley believes the key to clearing and keeping her skin clear has been eating lots of vegetables.

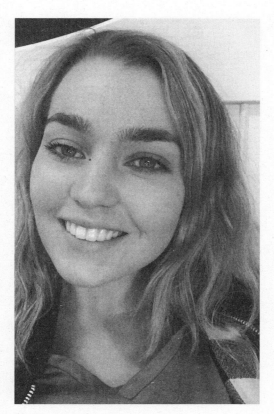

(See insert for color photos.)

2

ACNE ACTIVISTS: WHY US?

by Randa

"I mean, I had terrible, terrible, skin. It was embarrassing, and I did everything I could think of to make it go away. I tried to cover it with makeup. I tried to get rid of it with medication: oral, topical, even the harshest prescriptions. Nothing helped for very long."

—Film star Cameron Diaz[1]

While working on this book, Nina and I decided—along with our parents—to organize some Acne Intervention Programs in Los Angeles. We thought it would be beneficial to study people with acne in real life, rather than just relying on testimonials from social media to support the efficacy of the diet. When applying to be a participant in these programs, here is what some people told us about their acne:

- ❖ "I wake up in the morning and look in the mirror, and I'm disgusted by what I see."
- ❖ "Sometimes I want to leave school early, and I'll call my mom to come get me because my makeup is starting to come off and I can't stay there and be seen."
- ❖ "My acne changed me so much more than I thought would be possible."
- ❖ "My acne fills my mind with negative thoughts every day."
- ❖ "I avoid talking with other people because I'm afraid they'll be disgusted by looking at all the acne damage across my face."
- ❖ "I have tried everything to get rid of my acne. Nothing works."

❖ "I feel people are staring continuously at my face and that makes me very self-conscious."

❖ "I don't feel I'm attractive compared to other girls."

❖ "I was called 'pizza face' and 'non-Proactiv girl.'"

❖ "It got worse when my family started worrying about my face getting uglier every day."

❖ "It's gotten to the point where I don't leave my house anymore, other than to go to my job or walk my dog."

❖ "My acne makes me feel disgusting."

❖ "I think about my acne every second of every day."

❖ "I really have no more self-esteem."

❖ "It is something I am depressed by every day of my life."

❖ "I tried to kill myself because I could not handle the physical and emotional pain."

Practically all of this could have been written by me. To say "I totally relate" would be an understatement. These are the actual feelings the people applying for our Acne Intervention Programs expressed to us. The pain and the people are real.

When you think about it, as children we all take our faces for granted. Our skin is clear, smooth, unspoiled, radiant. We don't have to worry about what we look like—we just are who we are. But at some point, whether we like it or not, much of our self-esteem becomes linked to our appearance. Puberty hits, and the push to be attractive or perfect intensifies. And of course acne decides to inflict itself right when young people are emotionally most vulnerable.

Until Nina and I actually had bad acne ourselves, we didn't fully understand the extreme psychic misery so many teenagers and young adults were experiencing. The pain is both physical and mental. I've now done my time in the acne industrial complex, filled as it is with prescriptions and condescending advice that isn't very useful, like "Don't worry, you'll grow out of it" or "It could be worse" or "It's just normal, you're young" or "Stop picking your face, you're making it worse!" In the end, my sister and I came to the realization that we just don't live in a culture that is sufficiently supportive of acne sufferers.

It took getting slammed ourselves to fully comprehend the heartbreak created by this so-called rite of skin passage.

Acne woke us up.

CLEAR SKIN DIET PILOT STUDY

Why did Nina and I decide to do a series of acne interventions that ended up involving over 130 people? To answer that, you have to understand that living the clear skin lifestyle is a natural extension of our family's commitment to health. That commitment began when our mom got sick over twenty years ago. One day in 1995 our mom's ears turned red and started to blister and hurt. She thought that maybe she had gotten sunburned or was having an allergic reaction to shampoo. She first went to a dermatologist, who was very confused about her symptoms, and then bounced around to various doctors. Eventually, she found herself in the office of a noted rheumatologist who diagnosed her with a rare but serious autoimmune disease called relapsing polychondritis (RP).

No one knows what triggers RP. It's a disease where, in successive episodes over time, your immune system repeatedly attacks the cartilage in your body and destroys it. Because cartilage is not just around your ears, eyes, and nose but also around your throat and heart, RP is often life-threatening. According to one study, 40 percent of people who get the RP diagnosis that our mom got are dead in ten years.

While there's no known cure, the rheumatologist said he could help my mom "learn to live with it." That meant taking powerful drugs, some of which have serious side effects over time, including blindness.

Our mom decided to try something different and turned to the teachings of Dr. John McDougall. Dr. McDougall recommended using food to heal certain conditions, instead of prescription drugs.

Dr. McDougall was right. My mom's RP completely disappeared within weeks after she began following Dr. McDougall's dietary recommendations. Three months after changing her diet, her rheumatologist declared her RP in remission. My mom and dad were ecstatic. My parents continued eating along Dr. McDougall's guidelines to make sure my mom stayed healthy, and this is a major part of why my siblings and I were all raised on a vegan diet.

A FAMILY WITH A MISSION

Because my parents were grateful that my mom's life had been saved, they decided they wanted to help spread the word about the benefits of a healthy plant-based diet. In 1996, they opened a website called vegsource.com, calling it their form of "kitchen activism." Because our mom had changed her diet and dodged a bullet, our parents felt a duty to help others as they had been helped. Very quickly, they met and befriended many of the top medical experts, researchers, dietitians, and bestselling authors in the plant-based world. They coventured with many of these experts and worked hard to promote the experts' work on plant-based diets and health.

In 2001, my parents launched an annual health conference featuring top plant-based nutrition and medical experts. Nina and I grew up around some of the top plant-based doctors in the world, many of whom would stay in our home when they were in town.

Our parents also founded an all-volunteer nonprofit program, Meals for Health, which brings top plant-based experts into underserved communities for thirty-day immersion programs. The Meals For Health programs are free to participants. Typically, the programs are run in communities where there is a lot of heart disease, type 2 diabetes, hypertension, obesity, autoimmune diseases, and so on. The experts teach the hows and whys of a healthy plant-based diet, and it is an amazing and inspiring thing to behold. At the end of the month, nearly every participant's health has dramatically improved. Many no longer require their medications, have stabilized their vitals and lost weight, and feel better than they have in decades. Meals For Health programs change entire communities by proving to participants they can recover their health just by changing their diet.

When Nina and I witnessed followers on our social media trying our diet and freeing themselves of acne, a lightbulb went on. We believed there was another community that desperately needed a Meals For Health type of assistance—acne sufferers. We asked our parents if we could do a Meals For Health program featuring the Clear Skin Diet. We thought we could tailor the program to a younger crowd than Meals for Health normally serves—people with acne—and launch it here in Los Angeles. They agreed, and we were off and running.

CLINICAL PILOT STUDY OF CLEAR SKIN DIET

Our dad enlisted the help of Steve Lawenda, MD, a general practitioner at Kaiser Permanente Medical Group here in Los Angeles, who runs a very successful plant-based intervention program called Life 180. Dr. Lawenda is something of a medical hero around Kaiser in Southern California, with hundreds of patients clamoring to enroll in his programs in order to reverse their chronic diseases. Dr. Lawenda was the ideal doctor to supervise our pilot acne study.

Finding people in our online community with acne was not difficult at all. But recruiting people to take part in a free acne program turned out to be more challenging than we imagined. We went to the campus of a local university with a sign, flyers, and a clipboard to sign up people to receive more information by e-mail. The sign announced the program and had a before and after photos of Nina's acne.

If we had held up a "free weight loss program" sign with an impressive before and after photos, we probably would have been flooded with applicants. But people with severe acne who walked past us showed no interest. Some glanced quickly at our sign, then averted their eyes and hurried along like we weren't even there. We didn't want to stop anyone who had acne and say, "Hey, can I tell you about this program?" No one wants other people to bring up their acne. As people passed, Nina would just point to the photo of herself with acne and say "This was me, and this is me now." That attracted some interest, but it took some effort to get enough people to start our program. I think people were a little suspicious, wondering what we were selling.

There were fifteen participants in our first group, fifteen strangers whose curiosity had been piqued. They arrived on a sunny Southern California Saturday at a church meeting room we'd rented for the occasion. Eager and cautiously optimistic to learn how to get rid of their acne, they were equally skeptical. People with acne are leery of becoming too hopeful about a new cure; they've been failed so often in the past.

On the first Saturday of our program, we spent much of the day relating what we all called our "acne stories." We told ours; they told theirs; then we laid out the diet guidelines and shared some tips. Dr. Lawenda discussed the scientific side of acne and diet, and we brought in a professional chef to demonstrate how to make approved dishes.

We also gave them groceries. They received bags of potatoes, rice, oatmeal, whole wheat pasta, oil-free spaghetti sauce, salsa, corn tortillas, lentils...loads of healthy plant-based foods. We wanted it to be as easy as possible for them to start the diet immediately. Along with the food came the Clear Skin Diet program booklet, which included a meal plan and numerous easy recipes. Thereafter, we gathered every Tuesday night at the church. We'd eat a healthy meal and listen to a speaker, then have a roundtable discussion. It was incredibly comforting to be able to talk openly about how acne made each of us feel. We started joking about having formed the first acne support group ever.

Dr. Lawenda examined each participant at the beginning and again after thirty days and 'tracked participants during our weekly meetings. He documented the decrease in acne severity, lowered blood pressure, and weight loss. Our first acne intervention group lost a total of fifty pounds in the first thirty days, which was an average of over three pounds per person.

We started a second acne intervention group online, drawing from people all over the world. We created a private Facebook group, and the education was done using video live streaming. We had about 120 participants online. On the kickoff Saturday, Dr. Lawenda and the other experts came to our house, and we set up a mini studio in our family room. For several hours the speakers provided information about how and why the Clear Skin Diet works. The videos were available in the private Facebook group for everyone to watch.

Participants became more and more engaged after they started the diet and began to see their acne recede. The people from the first acne intervention group agreed to be coaches for the second group and shared their own tips, giving hope to people in the new group and inspiring them to "hang in there." The Facebook forum buzzed with hope, encouragement, and celebrations of each new success.

Results for some people came very quickly. Kendall Borys, Monika Marcinkiewicz, and Olivia all saw results in two weeks or less. You can see their dramatic before and after photos in the color insert in the middle of the book.

Kendall, age twenty, revealed she had started breaking out when she was sixteen. For four years she had been struggling with embarrassing and uncomfortable acne. "I'm so tired of getting acne," she wrote. "I get deep painful acne, and my face is bumps and mountains, which can make huge gaping holes! This scares me! And it leaves my skin insanely red with lots of discomfort." After starting the Clear Skin Diet, Kendall saw her face dramatically improve in less than two weeks (see Kendall's color photos in insert).

On seeing Kendall's results in only eleven days, our Meals For Health medical director Dr. Lawenda commented, "Many people wait eleven days just to see a dermatologist. Then, after waiting and finally seeing their dermatologist, they hear nothing about diet and are instead convinced to go on drugs, which they agree to do because they are feeling desperate. I am so happy for Kendall, and I'm blown away by the degree of participation in the group and the results! Frankly, the Clear Skin Diet is doing so much more for them than they would ever get from usual medical care."

Sixteen-year-old Monika said she started getting acne when she was eight, and nothing stopped the breakouts. After two weeks on the Clear Skin Diet, she reported: "Almost all my acne is gone! My skin is at its best state ever and I am so happy! I am shocked that I have not had a breakout on my forehead since I started, which has been the area that breaks out the most!" (See Monika's color photos in insert.)

Olivia also saw swift improvement when she started the program: "I've found taking photos has helped me so much and stopped me from giving up on this program because without it I think I would have been in denial about the sheer amount of progress I have been making with my skin. I've struggled with acne since I was eleven (I'm seventeen). Thank you to everyone involved in creating in this program! I'm honestly over the moon with my results so far and am filled with endless gratitude!" (See color photos in insert.)

Other Acne Intervention Program participants took longer to begin seeing benefits, like twenty-year-old Francesca Perticarini. Francesca was in our first acne intervention group, and at the end of the first thirty days, she didn't feel she had made enough improvement. Around week five or six though, she began to see significant results.

Maria DiGrazia joined the Acne Intervention Program after trying everything to get rid of acne on her arms. Nothing had worked. She had been taught that carbs were the enemy for weight loss, and she had been dieting on and off for years. She decided to give the program a try, and in less than six weeks, almost all of her arm acne was gone. See the color insert for photos of Francesca's and Maria's impressive transformations.

Not only did her acne clear, but Maria lost twenty pounds in those first six weeks—she was shocked, because she was enjoying the food and not holding back or trying to control what she ate. "I can't believe that I can eat as much as I want on this program and still lose weight!" she said. In five months, Maria lost a total of 40 pounds on the Clear Skin Diet. "I am sold on this program!"

Each participant in our Acne Intervention Program began with similar issues: acne severe enough to impact their lives, work, or school. For us, it underscores why acne needs to be viewed and treated more seriously. It's not "just acne." It's an epidemic, a sometimes soul-crushing disease. There are far too many people who feel hopeless about their acne and are largely ignored. Their suffering is treated as a "normal" part of growing up. It's not normal. It shouldn't be normal. It doesn't have to be.

DIET STOPS ACNE: KIRA LYNN MUKERJI, AGE 19

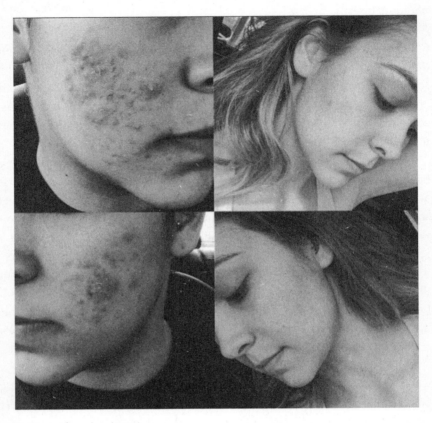

(See insert for color photos.)

Kira had severe cystic acne in high school and was "super embarrassed about it." She used heavy makeup and avoided social situations with bright lights. Kira tried everything, including going on birth control and Accutane, which cleared her acne completely. Unfortunately, once she stopped taking it, the acne came right back.

While browsing YouTube, Kira found our acne videos. She also read Dr. McDougall's writings on acne and decided to change her way of eating. Kira reported: "This diet worked incredibly well for me and cleared my skin. It has kept it clear for over a year!"

Kira says she now only gets a few small breakouts during her menstrual cycle, but they usually go away within a few days.

Kira also followed our recommendations for a more gentle skin-care approach and switched to gentle cleaners. Today, Kira doesn't use *any* face wash at all. "Before I changed my diet and my acne was raging, I would never have thought that using *no* face wash would help keep my skin be acne free! But the only thing I use on my face now is makeup remover wipes or water. Who would have thought!"

3

HOW FOOD TRIGGERS ACNE

by Nina

"Acne is a preventable disease, not a normal condition."

—John McDougall, MD

Randa and I had actually asked every dermatologist we met with whether diet could be playing a role in our breakouts. Although one did allow that dairy consumption could be a trigger for some people, the others seemed to agree that diet isn't a big factor for acne.

WHAT CAUSES ACNE?

I'm sure you're dying to learn more about acne, so here goes. Acne can take many forms—whiteheads, blackheads, pimples, and even large, cyst-like masses. Acne is the result of a hair follicle in your skin getting blocked. Skin cells constantly turn over. Old skin cells are shed every thirty days, and new ones are exposed. But if you're acne-prone and you have oily skin, the dead cells can get stuck.

Androgen hormones increase in both boys and girls during puberty, and these hormones can contribute to acne flares by overstimulating the sebaceous (oil) glands attached to the pores. The hormones provoke the release of sebum (oily matter) into your pores and onto your skin. Androgen hormones increase when you hit puberty or when you're stressed, making your oil glands kind of go crazy.

We all have a bacteria living on our skin called *Propionibacterium acnes (P. acnes)*. It's completely harmless—until it's fed with oil. When the *P. acnes* bacteria on your face has access to a plentiful oil supply, which your sebaceous glands pump out, it can inflame and infect the follicle. As the bacterial infection deepens and pressure grows behind the clogged pore, your immune system reacts, and a pus-filled bump forms on the top of your skin—a pimple. Acne is really the result of your skin trying to fight off infection, and the result is the undesirable big red zit.

ACNE AND CHOCOLATE—THE STUDY

When Randa and I were reading Dr. McDougall's articles during the drive to San Francisco, we were surprised to learn that very few experiments have been conducted on the possible relationship between food and acne. Dr. McDougall said one such study that had been given much weight was done back in the 1960s. It was commonly thought that chocolate caused acne. The Chocolate Manufacturers of America thought this was an unfortunate and false perception—not to mention bad for business. So they paid for a study on chocolate and acne. It was conducted by Dr. James Fulton and published in the *Journal of the American Medical Association* in 1969.[1]

Fulton took sixty-five young adults with bad acne and divided them into two groups. The first group was given a candy bar containing chocolate to eat every day, along with their regular diet. The second group got a nearly identical candy bar to eat each day, except the second group's candy bar did not contain any chocolate. At the end of four weeks, the kids in both groups had basically the same amount of acne as they did at the start of the study. From this, the researchers concluded that chocolate, and indeed diet in general, "has nothing to do with acne."

Note that the kids in both the chocolate and nonchocolate groups were eating candy bars that contained the same very high amounts of fat and sugar. That one candy bar had chocolate and the other did not was very likely irrelevant. This flawed chocolate candy bar study is one of just a tiny number of experiments published in the scientific literature attempting to test a specific food against acne.

WHERE NO ONE GETS ACNE

Most of the research on acne and diet comes from observational studies. Rather than testing specific foods for an acne response, researchers have looked at populations that have little or no acne to try to determine what patterns or associations may exist in those populations that might explain why acne isn't present.

For example, in 2002 a group of researchers from the United States, Sweden, and Australia joined to examine why acne was rampant in some societies while apparently nonexistent in others. They documented that in Westernized societies, acne is a nearly universal skin disease, afflicting 79 percent to 95 percent of the adolescent population and up to 54 percent of the population over age twenty-five. That means in places like the United States, Europe, and Australia, nearly everyone battles acne.

The researchers then looked at two non-Westernized populations where people had been eating their traditional diets for many generations. The researchers reported finding an "astonishing difference" in acne rates between the West and these non-Western populations. In the non-Western populations, researchers reported that acne was "completely absent"—not one person of the thousands they examined had ever had acne.

These acne-free individuals were from two distinct places: Papua New Guinea and Eastern Paraguay. Researchers reported that both groups lived primarily on unprocessed, low-fat plant foods—starches, vegetables, and fruits.[2] The Papua New Guinea study participants, for example, lived exclusively on root vegetables (yam, sweet potato, taro, tapioca), fruit (banana, papaya, pineapple, mango, coconut, guava, watermelon, pumpkin), vegetables, and fish. Researchers said the non-Western diets were very high in fiber and low in fat. The same researchers noted that South African Bantu children living on plant-food-based diets had an incidence of acne of only 16 percent, whereas Caucasians in wealthier Pretoria had an incidence of 45 percent—nearly three times higher.

The research in Papua New Guinea had been conducted in 1995 by Stefan Lindeberg, MD. Dr. Lindeberg studied 1,200 residents of a small island called Kitava. He found no acne in the 300 adolescents and young adults between the ages of fifteen and twenty-five he examined. If you assessed 300 American high school or college students, the majority would have acne—probably around 80 percent (or 240 of those 300 Americans). Yet according to Dr. Lindeberg's study, there was not one case of acne in anyone in Kitava—at any age. There was also virtually no obesity, heart disease, stroke, dementia, cancer, or high blood pressure either. Researchers noted the leading causes of death in Kitava occurred from malaria, drowning, and falling coconuts.

Another study, published in a dermatology journal in 1981, reported that people in rural Africa (Kenya and Zambia) who ate a plant-centered diet had little or no acne. The same researchers observed that for the Zulu tribes in South Africa, acne only became a problem when tribe members moved away from rural African villages to live in cities, where the food was much richer. They also noted research showing that Eskimos who adopted the Western diet after World War II "and probably as a result of the change to the Western diet" subsequently developed "a succession of new diseases"—including acne.[3]

Other researchers have published similar findings. In 1966, people from Malaysia living on rice-based diets were reported to have no acne problems.[4]

Researchers publishing in 1946 found that people in Okinawa, an isolated Japanese island in the South China Sea, had no acne vulgaris. Researchers reported the Okinawans ate a low-fat, starch-based diet comprised of 69 percent of calories from sweet potatoes and 88 percent of total calories from starch.[5] The same researchers noted that Europeans consuming lower-fat diets (such as in Crete and Southern Italy) were reported to have less acne compared to Western European countries where more fat is consumed. Yemenite Jews who followed a healthier, lower-fat diet than European Jews also reported less acne.[6]

All of these studies underscore one thing: while more than three out of four Americans eating the Western diet will get acne, among rural, non-Westernized people eating low-fat, high-fiber, starch-based diets, acne is virtually nonexistent. And in case you were thinking the non-Western populations were exercising more, which could influence acne, researchers reported physical activity levels were about the same between all groups studied and were not a factor.

WHAT ABOUT GENETICS?

Dr. Lindeberg's study of Kativans also found that genetics played little to no role in acne, noting that individuals who were genetically similar to the acne-free populations studied only became susceptible to Western illnesses or conditions when they moved and adopted a Western diet. Researchers observed that acne and other Western illness may be caused by diet and perhaps other environmental factors in the West but not by genetic predisposition. Clearly, some people can be more prone to acne than others. Two people can eat the same candy bar, and one person may break out while the other does not. But such predispositions to breakouts only seem to apply to people living in cultures where candy bars and other Western foods are regularly consumed. In those cultures where people eat a low-fat, starch-based diet, *no one* gets acne.

ACNE ADVICE:
From John McDougall, MD

The most unpalatable and unhealthy component of the American diet is grease—in other words, fats and oils. We wash our hands and face immediately when we get fats and oils on them. Strong detergents are used to remove grease from our countertops and walls. What do people call a restaurant with a bad reputation? A greasy spoon! The revulsion we feel toward grease is a way of protecting our health. The only way to make greasy foods palatable is to add salt, sugar, and spice to them—the more the better.

One reason manufacturers use fats and oils is to get the ingredients we do like to stick to our foods. Oils stick the salt to the potato chips and french fries, the sugar to the doughnuts, and the spices to the salad leaves. Fortunately, there are healthy ways for salt, sugar, and spice to stick to foods without using damaging fats and oils. We can easily remove grease from our diet by using nonstick cookware and healthy cooking and baking techniques. It's easy! And the food is even more delicious.

ACNE DRUGS VERSUS CHANGING YOUR DIET

Top acne researchers have uncovered evidence that the principle cause of acne is the Western diet. As we'll discuss in a moment, nearly all medications recommended by dermatologists to treat acne, including Accutane and Retin-A, work by trying to counteract the known acne-causing mechanisms of the Western diet.

When you realize that you're essentially being prescribed acne pills just so you can keep eating pizza and burgers, you need to ask yourself: Shouldn't I just change my diet in order to stop my acne? A recent research paper published in a major dermatology journal recommended exactly that.

The paper was published in *Dermato-Endocrinology*—a journal specializing in research on all aspects of investigation and clinical endocrinology of the skin. It urged dermatologists to educate patients about changing their diet, rather than simply giving drugs to treat symptoms. And the reasons to teach a healthier diet, according to these researchers, include the fact that the same unhealthy diet that promotes acne also promotes obesity, heart disease, cancer, type 2 diabetes, autoimmune diseases, and other common, chronic Western illnesses. It is not a coincidence that people with a history of severe teenage acne are more susceptible to developing certain cancers. For example, a recent study based on almost one hundred thousand women who were followed for over twenty years found those who had experienced severe teenage acne were 44 percent more likely to develop melanoma and 17 percent more likely to develop breast cancer, compared those with mild or no acne.[7] Another study of almost thirty-five thousand men found that those with a history of severe acne were significantly more likely to develop prostate cancer compared with men who'd had mild or no acne.[8]

This authoritative *Dermato-Endocrinology* paper pointing to a significant cause of acne was published in 2012 and looked at a particular enzyme in the body called mTORC1, which stands for mammalian target of rapamycin complex 1. This TOR enzyme plays a key role in promoting acne, according to this new research. When this TOR enzyme signaling goes up, acne occurs. So what causes this enzyme signaling to increase? The Western diet, according to the researchers. What foods specifically in the Western diet? The researchers are very specific: meat, dairy, junk food, high-fat, and highly refined foods—essentially the high-calorie, highly refined diet that most people consume in the West.[9] To raise your TOR enzyme, eat a turkey sandwich, ice cream, potato chips, or some oily pasta.

Researchers state flatly that TOR enzyme activity has produced "epidemic acne," and they said it drives "obesity, type 2 diabetes, cancer and neurodegenerative diseases." Fortunately, the researchers are very specific about how to combat acne: reduce (1) calories, (2) processed carbohydrates, (3) dairy products, and (4) animal products.

What is left, when you remove meat, dairy, and junky, fatty foods? The answer is the Clear Skin Diet.

The researchers say there is just one way to lower the acne-causing TOR enzyme, and that is: "by increasing the consumption of vegetables and fruit." The paper strongly urges dermatologists to advise patients to change their diets away from a Western diet "not only to improve acne" but also to avoid developing diabetes, heart disease, cancer, and other chronic diseases later in life.

I mentioned at the start of this section that recent research suggests that all of the popular anti-acne medications are now thought to work by inhibiting this TOR enzyme activity. These drugs are trying to combat what are side effects of the foods most people in the West chose to eat. Researchers report that

Accutane, benzoyl peroxide, Retin-A, a range of antibiotics such as doxycycline, tetracyclines, and erythromycin all are now thought to work against acne by directly or indirectly attenuating TOR enzyme signaling.[10] But of course none of these anti-acne drugs actually addresses the underlying problem of why the TOR enzyme was elevated in the first place—your diet. And these drugs are, at best and when they work, temporary fixes. Some carry potentially serious side effects. Adopting the Clear Skin Diet and eliminating the foods that cause TOR enzyme elevation is the drug-free solution to the problem.

If you had fires regularly breaking out at your house, would you address the problem with a special sprinkler system that turned on every time a new fire started? Or would you want to find out *why* the fires were starting, and then address *that* issue in order to stop the fires from breaking out in the first place? That is essentially the choice between using drugs and medicine to battle breakouts versus making critical changes to your diet to simply make the acne go away.

The conclusion of the *Dermato-Endocrinology* paper reiterates that dermatologists "should take responsibility for dietary education" of their patients in order to stop acne. The researchers write that a deeper understanding of the TOR enzyme as the cause of acne and the ability of a healthy diet to stop it will help the dermatologist "to appreciate the statement of Hippocrates of Kós who said about 2,400 years ago, 'Your diet should be your medicine, and your medicine should be your diet.'"

WHY A LOW-FAT DIET?

A crucial aspect of the Clear Skin Diet is that it is very low in fat. Does that freak you out? I hope not! I'm going to explain why lowering your fat intake is so important. The Clear Skin Diet has been crafted to replicate as closely as possible the dietary parameters of the acne-free cultures we've discussed. While the standard American diet gets about 35 percent of calories from fat, the Clear Skin Diet gets around 10 percent of calories from fat. Now when professionals in the United States talk about a low-fat diet, they are usually referring to a diet containing 25 to 30 percent of calories from fat—really not that much lower than the 35 percent most people already eat.

The 10 percent of calories from fat in the Clear Skin Diet is often referred to by professionals as "extremely" low fat, in effect dismissing it. Who wants to eat an extreme diet? In fact, it is the modern high-fat, junky, high-calorie Western diet that is extreme. According to T. Colin Campbell, PhD, author of *The China Study*, and professor emeritus of Nutritional Biochemistry at Cornell University, a whole food, plant-based diet, without added oil and refined carbohydrates, has the greatest ability to restore and maintain health. This diet is "fashioned over millions of years by nature and its nutritional composition just so happens to be about 10–12% fat, 10–12% protein and 75–80% carbohydrates, while being chocked full of life-promoting antioxidants and the right kinds and ratios of fats, proteins and carbohydrates."

The Clear Skin Diet is powered by foods that humans have eaten for millennia. The populations studied in Kenya, Malaysia, Paraguay, Okinawa, and Malaysia—where acne doesn't exist—ate somewhere between 6 and 10 percent of their calories from fat. The populations that eat this low-fat diet not only avoid acne, heart disease, and obesity, but they also acquire something else: longevity. They live significantly longer than other cultures in the world. And they don't just live longer, they live in better health to the very end of their lives. They don't need wheelchairs or have to be warehoused in assisted-living facilities when they get old. After a long life of ninety or one hundred years, their good diet and lifestyle habits have left them in very good shape.

THE BLUE ZONES

Researchers looking at longevity often focus on areas where a significant percentage of people have reached the age of one hundred or more and are still in optimal health. You may have heard of Blue Zones, which refer to populations in the world with unusually high concentrations of healthy centenarians. Okinawa is a Blue Zone and has some of the longest-lived people on the planet (in addition to having great skin).

To be considered a Blue Zone, scientists must first validate that the people are actually as old as they claim; it's not always possible to get reliable records from a hundred years ago. And while it's possible to measure what centenarians are eating now, what did they eat before, which allowed them to reach the one-hundred-year mark?

The Okinawan islands in Japan turn out to have a wealth of well-documented historical information. Researchers have validated the birthdates on record for nearly all Okinawan centenarians—of whom there are many. Then, because the local Okinawan government conducted detailed population surveys starting in 1949, researchers have been able to obtain detailed information on the composition of their diet over many years.

The healthiest and longest-lived centenarians basically ate the Clear Skin Diet:

OKINAWAN DIET—1949

TYPE OF FOOD	PERCENT OF TOTAL CALORIES
Sweet potatoes	69%
Rice	12%
Other grains	7%
Legumes	6%
Other vegetables	3%
Oils	2%
Fish	1%
Nuts, seeds, sugar, meat, eggs, dairy, fruit, alcohol	Combined less than 1%

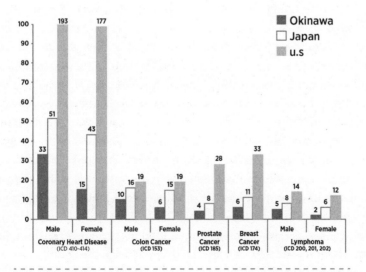

FIGURE 5. Mortality from age-associated diseases in Okinawans versus Americans. Numbers represent age-adjusted mortality rate in deaths per hundred thousand persons per year for 1995. Coding was according to ICD-9 codes. Populations were age-adjusted to World Standard Population. These data show markedly lower mortality risk from age-related diseases in Okinawans versus other Japanese and Americans.

Except for the trivial amounts of oil, fish, meat, and nuts that Okinawans consumed (less than 4 percent of total calories), an Okinawan-style diet derives about 88 percent of its calories from carbohydrates (sweet potatoes, rice, and other grains). People who eat within these guidelines don't get acne when they are teens, and they don't develop the diseases that cause premature deaths in the West. The chart on the preceding page comes from one of the Okinawan longevity studies. It shows some common diseases and the incidence per hundred thousand persons for each of the three areas—Okinawa, Japan, and the United States. As you can see, the Okinawans have but a fraction of these diseases, compared to the other populations:[11]

The chart indicates that women in the United States have twelve times more incidences of heart disease and six times more breast cancer than women in Okinawa. It's worth repeating that the same diet that heals your skin can prevent or reverse many other serious Western diet–inflicted diseases.

OIL IS JUST LIQUID FAT

On the Clear Skin Diet you'll be removing all vegetable oil from your diet, whether it's canola, soybean, corn, sunflower, olive, coconut, peanut, or any other kind of oil (including, of course, fish oil).

Oil in its simplest form is not a natural food; it's a highly processed food. You only get it by taking an actual food, like a whole olive, squeezing out all of the fat, and putting it in a bottle. Meanwhile, you have removed the protein, fiber, carbohydrates, and nutrients like vitamins and minerals. Normally, when you eat a plant, like corn, olives, or coconut, you get fiber, carbohydrates, nutrients, protein, and fat—all in the right amounts. The food enters your mouth, stomach, bloodstream, and cells all in perfect harmony. When that small amount of fat contained in the food enters your cells, it is combined with the right amount of other nutrients. Thus, you get everything for health from your whole food—as nature intended.

But when you extract the fat from a food and create a separate bottle of pure fat, you have isolated, concentrated, and changed the nature of that food. You now have a substance that is super calorie dense; oil contains 9 calories per gram, whereas sugar and animal protein have 4 calories per gram, and starch has only 1 calorie per gram. A pound of olive oil contains a whopping 4,000 calories. A pound of refined sugar, on the other hand, has "just" 1,725 calories. And a pound of potatoes is about 400 calories. Oil is an overly processed, calorie-dense substance that can make you quickly gain unwanted weight and unwanted acne.

When you consume this concentrated fat (oil), it moves very quickly through your stomach and bloodstream into your cells where it is easily stored as fat. It means these calorie-dense fats are easily stored in your body and help you gain or retain weight. You will be "wearing" this fat on your face, when some of it naturally leeches out onto your skin's surface.

Vegetable oils are a relatively new addition to the human diet. The current prevalent use of oils added into foods was practically nonexistent before 1900. Oil consumption has doubled since 1980, coinciding with the increased consumption of meat and dairy. In short, most people living in the West switched to a very high fat diet in only the past one hundred years or so, and the results in terms of acne, obesity, and health in general have been devastating.

DAIRY EQUALS ACNE JUICE

Here is something kind of gross to think about. Fat isn't the only thing that contributes to acne. Of course our hormones play a big part. High-fat, high-animal-product diets can promote hormone changes. There is a protein called insulin-like growth factor 1 (IGF-1). IGF-1 is raised when you eat dairy and meat and other high-protein animal foods. IGF-1 is also pimple food. Research has shown that higher IGF-1 blood levels have an effect promoting acne and making acne more severe, especially in women.[12] Overall, the rich Western diet elevates the same sex hormones that stimulate acne.

The connection between milk consumption and severe acne is widely confirmed in recent research. One study used data from the Harvard Nurses Health Study II and found that dairy drinkers had more acne than nondairy drinkers. Why? The researchers wrote: "We hypothesize that the association with milk may be because of the presence of hormones and bioactive molecules in milk." That makes sense, since dairy is a high-fat food. But hold on! The same study also showed that people consuming skim milk (fat-free dairy) actually had *more* acne and more severe acne than those consuming whole, full-fat milk.[13]

Now why would milk with no fat cause even more acne than milk with lots of fat? Again, it may be the hormones. Our own hormones during adolescence trigger sebum production on our face, and it turns out skim milk contains the highest levels of total hormones, compared to 2 percent or whole milk.[14] Why this is hasn't been fully explained. It may be that when you skim off all the fat from milk, you are leaving behind more concentrated levels of IGF-1. The fat acts to dilute those substances in whole milk, but fat-free milk may contain even more concentrated hormones by volume. Hormones in milk are designed to make a calf grow, and grow quickly. Dairy products—cheese, ice cream, milk—stimulate growth generally, and research suggests they can stimulate acne in many people.

WHAT ABOUT MEAT AND OIL IN THE OKINAWAN DIET?

The Okinawans were not 100 percent plant based; they ate a small amount of fish and pork, as well as oil. Why would Okinawans be acne- and heart disease-free if they were eating these foods? It turns out the Okinawans didn't eat very much pork at all, and they didn't eat it very often, just on certain holidays. They also boiled and stewed their pork for three days, cooking out and skimming off the fat. What they ate in the end was the high-protein collagen and very little pork fat.

You may ask, "Why doesn't the Clear Skin Diet also allow a very small bit of oil or animal foods?" Everything in moderation, right? And the answer is the Clear Skin Diet is 100 percent plant-based because it's easier that way. Eating just a small, measured amount of animal products or high-calorie foods can

ACNE ADVICE:
From Alona Pulde, MD

Do you ever get dark circles under your eyes when you are tired? Blush pink or red when you are anxious, excited, or embarrassed? Become pale when you are scared or not feeling well? Glow when you are feeling elated or happy? Then you may well understand how our skin is often a window to our health and well-being. And although it is true that beauty is not only skin deep, the state of our skin certainly contributes to our beauty currency. Remember your skin is the window to your health and well-being. As such, eating well and having a healthy inside will also make for a healthier outside. By far, the most important contributor to healthy skin is your diet. And more specifically, your diet of low-fat, whole plant-based foods. The more fruits, vegetables, whole grains, and legumes that you can add to your diet, the more water, fiber, vitamins, and minerals you are consuming. This nutritional jackpot helps to eliminate the toxins you don't want while holding on to the hydrating and nourishing nutrients you do want.

be difficult. If we recommended just a little meat like the Okinawans, maybe a few ounces a week, people would probably end up eating much more than that. If you came home late and were hungry and there was a roast chicken in your fridge, and you were only supposed to eat a few ounces of it, you might think, "Well, I'm starving, nothing else is ready, so I might as well finish it off. Just this once." So much for "moderation." It doesn't work for most people. Moderation for one person might mean a binge for someone else. Keeping temptation around and encouraging minute portions is a recipe for failure. Moderation in practice can actually be harder than total avoidance.

Another good reason to ignore the whole "moderation" concept is that if you eat just *some* higher fat foods, your taste buds may not adjust to your new diet as quickly as they otherwise would. When you first embark on the Clear Skin Diet, you might temporarily miss some of the fatty foods you're accustomed to. Your brain rewards you with a big, fat dopamine hit, a chemical that signals pleasure, whenever you consume foods high in calories, sugar, salt, and fats. These dopamine hits can make unhealthy foods become literally addictive. But when you leave that food behind completely, after a short time your taste buds adjust, and healthy plant-based foods start to taste amazing. Healthy food tastes wonderful once you wean yourself off less healthy foods.

—◇—

DIET STOPS ACNE: BRIAN TURNER, AGE 24

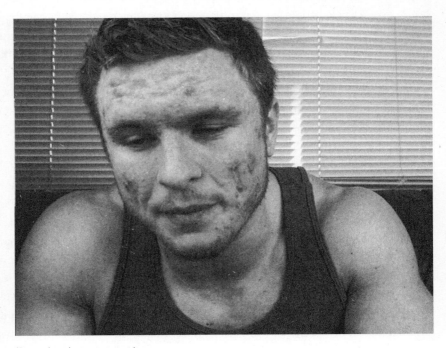

(See color photos in insert.)

At fifteen years old, Brian started getting acne, which soon began developing very large nodular cysts. The cysts would refuse to heal for months, and he would have three or four at a time. Brian's acne grew increasingly severe over the years, to the point where his face was completely covered: "My entire face felt pressurized. People who have actually dealt with severe acne know what I'm talking about. Your whole face is so painful that even lying down on a pillow hurts."

Brian was on Accutane for seventy weeks. It took nearly a year for it to begin working. His skin got so dry that sometimes if he laughed or smiled too hard, the skin around the corners of his mouth would crack and bleed. Then the Accutane stopped working, and his acne returned. Brian tried everything and found only one thing that worked—a plant-based diet. Brian removed animal products from his diet, starting with dairy. He began to regularly hydrate and eat lots of vegetables. "As I ate more and more servings of vegetables every day, crowding out other foods I might normally eat, I found my skin just got better and better. I got to a point where I eat between ten to sixteen servings

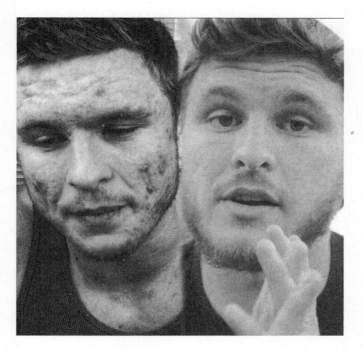

of vegetables a day, and my acne became completely under control. It worked better than Accutane."

Brian had struggled with severe acne for nine years and was bullied relentlessly at times. Now he feels grateful for the experience; he teaches others about using a vegan diet to stop acne and how to effectively remove acne scars. In fact, Brian works with us and was one of the instructors in our clear skin Acne Intervention Programs.

4

INTRODUCING THE CLEAR SKIN DIET

by Randa

"This diet is literally magic. I am in awe that in only one week my skin is looking like this. ONE WEEK!"

—Kendall Borys, Acne Intervention Program participant

I am certain you are eager to have a new and improved relationship with your skin. This chapter is going to explain what you're going to eat and what you're going to avoid.

Once you know what foods to eat and have translated those foods into your favorite meals and dishes, you will be on the way to eradicating your acne.

WHAT TO EAT?

The secret to the success of the Clear Skin Diet shouldn't be a secret at all. It just means eating like the people of Kenya, Malaysia, Paraguay, Okinawa, and the rest of the places where research has shown acne does not exist. Adolescents and young adults in these populations may have stressful lives and other problems that everyone deals with, but acne is not one of them. Eat like they do, and you can eliminate your own acne.

Each of these populations eats a diet based on the food locally available. But the overall composition of their diets is very similar.

There are so many amazing-tasting acne-busting foods you'll learn to love. So let's get started on your journey.

THE CLEAR SKIN DIET GUIDELINES

Here are the six pillars of the Clear Skin Diet:

1. Plant foods only, no animal products
2. Unrefined starches should be the cornerstone of your diet
3. Avoid all oils
4. Avoid high-fat plant foods
5. Eat *whole* foods, food as grown, minimally processed
6. Eat simply; variety is not important, repetition can promote long-term success

Let's take a look at each guideline in more detail.

1. PLANT FOODS ONLY—WE'RE NOT KIDDING

Your diet will be comprised of foods from plant origin only. No meat (beef, lamb, pork, venison), no poultry (chicken, turkey, duck), no fish or shellfish, no eggs, no dairy products (milk, cheese, butter), and no animal-derived ingredients (like casein or whey).

Instead, you will focus on whole grains, legumes, fruits, and vegetables.

2. MAKE UNREFINED STARCH THE FOCUS OF YOUR DIET

Starches are low in fat, low in calories, and high in satiation (meaning starches make you feel full and satisfied). You are going to be eating comfort foods like rice, potatoes, breads, pastas, beans, corn, sweet potatoes, and oatmeal. One of our Acne Intervention Program participants, Maria DiGrazia, was pleasantly surprised to learn that she was "allowed" to eat potatoes. "This is the first meal I've eaten in a long time without shame," she exclaimed, while eating a stuffed baked potato at our first meeting. People are almost relieved to hear that they can have starchy foods again. These complex delicious carbohydrates will end up being the cornerstone of your diet—perhaps 70 to 80 percent of your calories and even more in some cases. The rest will be other vegetables and fruits.

A great way to succeed on the Clear Skin Diet is to pinpoint your favorite starch-based meal. You can even have the same dish for every meal, like eating potatoes for breakfast, lunch, and dinner.

ACNE ADVICE:
From John McDougall, MD

The secret to a successful diet is to center it around delicious, satisfying starches. Everyone remembers these "comfort foods" that we loved growing up—potatoes, rice, pastas, corn, beans, oatmeal, and whole grains. Starches are high in complex carbohydrates and dietary fiber, very low in fat, and contain no cholesterol. They are loaded with vitamins and minerals and always contain generous amounts of healthy vegetable protein that satisfies the nutritional needs of growing children and adults. Fruits and yellow and green vegetables are important additions to a starch-centered meal plan, providing a cornucopia of color, flavor, texture, and aroma, as well as additional nutrients.

Don't be fooled into believing that all carbs make you fat. It's just not true. Unrefined starches are only about one calorie per gram (which is extremely low) and have been the cornerstone of healthy, trim populations throughout history. Think rice in Asia, potatoes in South America, sweet potatoes in Papua New Guinea, wheat and barley in the Middle East, and corn and beans in Mexico. It is only when these populations detoured from their local diets and started consuming unfamiliar meats, dairy, oils and processed foods that they began experiencing weight and health issues.

3. AVOID ALL OILS

Avoid all vegetable oils, such as olive, corn, safflower, canola, flaxseed, and coconut oil. What, no coconut oil? Isn't that healthy? *No!* All oils are 100 percent fat, including coconut oil. That fat can be delivered straight to your face. Avoid any packaged foods that may contain oil. Avoiding oil means avoid all margarines (such as Earth Balance, Smart Balance, Can't Believe It's Not Butter), avoid all fake meats or fake cheeses (veggie dogs, veggie sausages, veggie burgers, veggie lunch meats, veggie ice creams, vegan cheese), and check labels in order to avoid any food that lists oil as an ingredient; see chapter 11 on label reading.

4. AVOID HIGH-FAT PLANT FOODS

Avoid all high-fat plant foods including nuts, nut butters (such as peanut butter, including reduced fat peanut butter, almond butter, cashew butter), all seeds, olives, coconuts, and avocados (such as found in guacamole). Nuts contain be-tween 80 and 90 percent of calories from fat, seeds are about 70 to 75 percent calories from fat, olives are 80 percent calories from fat, coconuts are about 85 percent calories from fat, and avocados are up to 88 percent of calories from fat. Your face doesn't want this fat.

Avoid any products that contain any of these foods as ingredients—nuts, seeds, olives, coconut, or avocado.

Avoid soy products, as well as soy milk and other plant milks unless they are 100 percent fat-free (you can make your own oat milk—see "Bonus Recipes" in the Recipes section). Avoid soy-based or tofu-based foods (which are high in fat). Avoid vegan packaged fake burgers, vegan energy bars (unless 100 percent fruit), hummus (unless low-fat and made without oil or seeds like tahini), and other processed vegan foods.

Don't be fooled into thinking that just because a food has a vegan label that it is health food. These higher fat processed foods are not health promoters—they are acne promoters. We will show you how to make your own tasty burgers (see Recipes), but you don't need any store-bought, premade, processed vegan foods.

Let's take a second to answer a question that usually comes up about now. And that question is: "Am I going to stop eating nuts, seeds, coconuts, avoca-dos, and so on for the rest of my life?" And the answer is: you will not be eating these foods while you are in the process of halting the progression of your acne and healing your skin. For some people, this can happen very quickly on the Clear Skin Diet; for others it may take a number of months. Once your acne has cleared, you can experiment if you would like with adding these types of foods

ACNE ADVICE:
From Matthew Lederman, MD

Although jumping in 100 percent to a lower-fat, whole food, plant-based diet will get you results most quickly, some people don't have to be 100 percent strict to still get significant results. The problem is that, at first, you don't know that you are one of those people. If you are not, then doing the program 90 percent might not get you to the finish line. I recommend jump-ing in 100 percent for twelve weeks just to see what your body can actually do and the results you can actually achieve. After you've accomplished your goals, you can start to test whether you want to add back some "less ideal" foods to your diet, if any.

back into your diet, one at a time. This is like a reverse-elimination diet. We eliminate most all acne trigger foods to clear your face. Once your face is clear, you can add these foods one at a time back for a week or two, if that's what you want to do, and see whether your acne returns—you'll usually find out pretty quickly whether or not it's a trigger food. But until you have tamed your acne, you are going to stay the heck away from higher fat plant foods.

5. EAT WHOLE FOODS

Focus your diet on whole foods and minimally processed foods. Spend most of your shopping time in the produce department of your supermarket, not the packaged food area. A whole food is a food that has been processed or refined as little as possible—a food that looks like it came off a tree or bush or out of the ground—and doesn't have anything added to it. Avoid refined foods like white rice, white flour, white bread, white pasta, and any other processed foods— cakes, cookies, potato chips, soft drinks, doughnuts. These are all examples where parts of the original food were processed out, leaving only some of the original food, and thus they aren't whole foods. (Some of these processed foods may actually be permitted, but only when they are homemade and prepared according to the guidelines—see Recipes.) When you eat bread, for example, it should be whole wheat. Whole is an important factor when buying foods because it means the food is less processed and minimally processed is better for you (see chapter 11 for label-reading tips).

An example of a minimally processed food is oatmeal. The grains of the oat plant (called oat groats) are either ground up (sometimes called milled oats) or rolled (rolled oats). While you are not eating the whole oat as grown, the processing to the oats in this case has been minimal. A potato chip, on the other hand, is generally created using a dough made from dehydrated potatoes, which is then pressed into a desired shape. Chemicals or other ingredients may be added, the chip is then deep fried in oil or other fat, salted, and placed into an airtight container. Potato chips are an example of a highly processed, very acne-promoting food. It's a shame to treat a perfectly nice potato that way!

6. EAT SIMPLY

The final guideline is that, when you find a meal you like, eat it over and over again. Don't worry about whether you are getting enough of this vitamin or that nutrient. As long as you are eating an unrefined diet based around starch, with fruit and/or green and yellow vegetables on occasion, you're getting everything your body requires.

ACNE ADVICE:
From Jeff Novick, MS, RD

Keep food choices as simple as possible and resist every influence to make them complicated. You don't need five versions of oatmeal, fifteen dinners, fancy pots, pans, utensils, and so on. All you need are some simple basics, such as oatmeal, brown rice, beans, and a few veggies and fruits that you like. They don't have to be organic, non-GMO, fair-trade, imported, or any of that. They can be fresh, they can be frozen, they can be canned—whichever makes it easiest. Instead of looking for imported Japanese *satsuma* sweet potatoes, just eat any potatoes you can find.

You may discover an item you like and are willing to eat consistently for any given meal—oatmeal or hash browns for breakfast, beans and rice or a big baked potato with toppings for lunch. Find a handful of dishes that you like and eat these meals again and again and again. Make them in large batches and store them in your fridge or freezer so you can fire up a meal of leftovers on short notice.

SO WHAT'S LEFT?

Now you've read the six guidelines, and you might be thinking: That's a lot of no's, what about some yes's? Well, don't feel intimidated. There are still so many foods available to you. And remember: you're not restricting food intake, you're restricting acne outbreaks! Here is just a partial list of the delicious foods you'll discover on the Clear Skin Diet.

For breakfast: oatmeal with fruit, pancakes, cold cereal (with fat-free plant milk), hash brown potatoes, French toast, waffles.

For lunch and dinner (or breakfast): potatoes (baked, boiled, steamed, mashed with gravy), bean soups, lentil soups, bread, sweet potatoes, lasagna, brown rice, pizza, spaghetti, burritos, noodles, beans, corn, stir-fries, veggie sushi, salads with barley, couscous, maize, millet, bean burgers, sandwiches, fruits, vegetables, and sauces, dips, salt, sugar, and spices.

And for dessert, you can have brownies or fruit, banana smoothie "ice cream," pudding, or sorbet.

ACNE ADVICE:
From Neal Barnard, MD

If making these changes seems like a tall order, don't worry! It's easier than you think. Pick a day to start when you focus on succeeding. Avoid beginning when you're traveling a lot or have deadlines at school or work. Then set a goal of giving it 100 percent. That will allow your body to enjoy the healthiest foods on the planet—and help you see great results.

MAKING IT WORK

We want to share additional thoughts and tips to help assure success for your Clear Skin Diet program. In our successful Acne Intervention Programs, we encourage participants to keep a food journal and record everything they eat and drink, other than water. Many of them found tracking beneficial. You might simply write down the name of a recipe, if you use one from this book. But otherwise, note everything you consume and generally try to do so right after each meal or snack. Some intervention participants kept their food journal in a booklet, others wrote it as a note on their phones, and some used a free app like MyNetDiary. The point is not to track calories or macros but to become aware of what exactly you're eating. If you're not getting results as fast as you would like, you will have a record of all your food, and you can talk about it with others including on the Clear Skin Diet discussion forums.

Also, over time you may begin to see specific food sensitivities. If you start having a breakout at a certain point, you can look at what you were eating the day or days right before that happened to see if you can identify a trigger food. Also, later when your acne has subsided, you may be curious about whether a specific food makes you break out. The way to do that, once you're clear, is to introduce that food back into your diet, just that one food. For example, maybe you want to have some oil-free hummus, which is higher fat because it contains tahini (ground sesame seeds). You could try it, write down how much you had, and then see if there is an acne effect over the next few days. When testing food sensitivities, keeping a record of what you're eating is critical.

DRINK WATER

The foods in the Clear Skin Diet contain a higher water content than most people may be accustomed to eating, and the added water is a bonus. Increased water consumption could be helpful in resolving breakouts. While your thirst is the best indicator of the amount of water you need, we do recommend making a conscious effort to drink more water, at least during the initial period of the program. Although there isn't much in the way of formal research indicating that drinking more water is going to help fight acne, we do know that water boosts blood flow and can help clear toxins.

Fellow acne activist Brian Turner, whose story was at the end of the last chapter, credits increasing his water intake as one of the keys for curing his severe cystic acne.

ACTUALLY GET A GOOD NIGHT'S SLEEP

Easier said than done, we know. According to the National Sleep Foundation, teens require at least eight to ten hours of sleep a night to function at their best, but they get an average of seven. One study found that only 15 percent of teens reported sleeping eight and a half hours on school nights. Chronic sleep deprivation can have a serious impact on the physical, mental, and behavioral health of a young adult. They're not getting enough sleep during a time when they need it most. Early classes, tons of homework, exams, social pressures, extracurricular activities—who has time to sleep?

There is research suggesting that sleep deprivation can cause acne. One study found that the risk of psychological stress increases by 14 percent by each hour of sleep you miss each night. Stress increases glucocorticoid production, which dermatologists say can lead to abnormalities in skin structure and function.

What can you do to get more sleep? Make an effort to go to bed earlier. Using the hour before sleep as quiet time can help. Try to make your room as dark as possible, as even a small amount of light can interfere with your sleep. Avoid intense exercise before bed, and stay away from bright artificial light like your TV, phone, or computer screen. This light can signal your brain that it is time to be awake and slow production of hormones that would help you fall asleep.

STOP BEING A STRESS BALL

Some dermatologists believe inflammation can be promoted by stress. School is stressful. Perhaps you have a particularly demanding work schedule and are staying up late, worrying about completing projects. Or maybe you've just experienced a breakup, and now you're breaking out. Researchers at Stanford University found that students had increased acne flare-ups during exam periods, compared to times when they weren't being tested. Scientists don't know exactly how stress impacts acne, but if you are feeling anxious, think about ways to take action. Maybe review your schedule and look for ways to give yourself more time to finish projects, learn new relaxation exercises, talk to a professional—be aware that finding ways to destress can help your complexion.

EXERCISE

One of the best stress relievers is exercise. It can improve sleep, lower stress, and keep your blood circulation pumping, which sends more oxygen to skin cells and helps carry away waste. The benefits of exercise are so colossal, we have an entire chapter about it ahead (see chapter 15).

DITCH THE CAFFEINE

You may love your morning joe or friendly cup of tea. We do too. Neither of us have ever been coffee drinkers, but there was a point in our lives when we were sipping (OK, guzzling) tea all day long. Coincidentally, our tea drinking habit coincided with our acne breakouts.

We do suggest that you stop drinking caffeinated drinks during the initial months of the Clear Skin Diet program. You may have to go caffeine-free while your skin is healing for some number of months. Although there isn't definitive research tying caffeine to acne, coffee is acidic and could influence hormones and blood sugar. Caffeine can also impact your stress levels by affecting your sleep. Caffeine in larger amounts could potentially dehydrate your skin, which you want to avoid.

DITCH THE ALCOHOL

We know, Nina and Randa are total party poopers. Alcohol too? *What?!* Remember that your skin is a reflection of your overall health, so we want to encourage health-promoting behavior. Although it's not been proven that alcohol directly causes acne, alcohol can impact hormone levels and cause an imbalance of testosterone or estrogen levels that can contribute to acne. Your liver helps clear toxins from your body, and alcohol can, in significant amounts over time, reduce your liver function. Alcohol can also be dehydrating. Regular indulgence in alcohol can depress your immune system, which also isn't conducive to acne-free skin. So we recommend you quit drinking entirely while you are getting your acne under control.

DITCH THE SMOKING

Obviously, there are absolutely no health benefits associated with cigarette smoking. As far as acne is concerned, nine studies have looked at whether there is a connection between acne and smoking. Three seemed to indicate that smoking actually *improved* acne; four pointed toward smoking contributing negatively to acne; and two were inconclusive. That said, there is no debate about whether smoking is harmful to your skin (not to mention your health!). Smoking slows the healing process, meaning that your acne will stay active for longer periods; it causes wrinkles and premature aging (nothing like having acne *and* wrinkles!); it stains the teeth and makes your hair fall out. If you want to heal your acne in order to improve your appearance, then you definitely want to quit smoking too.

BEWARE OF OILY SUPPLEMENTS

One of the participants in our Acne Intervention Programs wasn't seeing results as quickly as she was hoping. She said she was adhering to the diet religiously, but her acne was still active. She carefully scrutinized everything that came into contact with her face and everything she was putting into her mouth. And then she discovered that she actually *had* been consuming oil but from a surprising source. She was taking a vitamin D supplement, which contained oil. She discontinued the supplement, and within a few weeks her acne began to recede impressively. She believed that the very small amount of daily oil contained in a soft-gel pill was the difference between having new breakouts and healing her acne.

SUGAR SUGAR

Fat is implicated far more in acne than sugar, although the combination of sugar and fat—aka junk food—is probably the worst of all worlds. But some people may have particular sugar sensitivities. If you have been following the Clear Skin Diet for a couple of months and are looking to improve your results, try eliminating any added sugars. Plain white sugar is just a refined sweetener; eliminate it along with syrup, corn syrup, and cane juice and see how this impacts your acne.

—◇—

The Clear Skin Diet Cheat Sheet

Diet Guidelines

Plant foods only
Unrefined starches should be the cornerstone of your diet
Avoid all oils
Avoid high-fat plant foods
Eat *whole* foods, food as grown, less processed
Eat simply, repeat things you like

Tips to Consider

Drink water
Get sleep
Destress
Exercise
Ditch caffeine

Ditch alcohol
Ditch smoking
Beware of hidden oil
Don't go overboard on
processed sugar

—◇—

DIET STOPS ACNE: DANI STOUGH, AGE 16

Dani Stough said she started having acne fifteen months before applying to be a participant in one of our acne immersion programs. In her application e-mail, Dani wrote: "I can't get my acne to go away! I just don't know what to do anymore!"

Dani found her acne starting to fade in just ten days after starting the Clear Skin Diet:

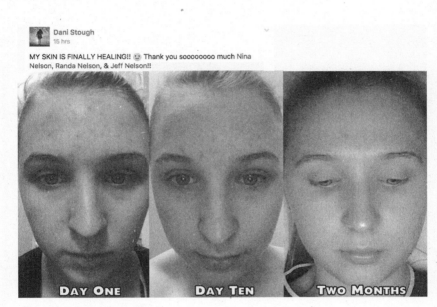

(See color photos in insert.)

Later Dani posted in the Facebook group about her experimenting to see whether it was in fact the Clear Skin Diet curing her acne:

THANK YOU SOOOO MUCH!! 😊 😊 😊 I just had to say that because you changed my life!! I started this diet on June 25th and by July 5th (10 days) my face was pretty much clear. Then I wanted to be certain that not eating oil or overt fats, was what was healing it rather than something else... so I purposefully had some avocado and had a dish with oil in it (July 7th)... the next day my face had 4 new pimples, and was red and inflamed. That is when I knew it was the fats and oil. So OF COURSE, I stopped eating all that stuff 6 days ago (July 9th). MY FACE IS ALMOST COMPLETELY CLEAR AGAIN!! So... THANK YOU SOOOO MUCH to everyone but especially... Nina Nelson, Randa Nelson, & Jeff Nelson!!! 😊 😊 😊

5

FOOD FACTS AND FICTIONS

by Randa

"A healthy diet is a solution to many of our health-care problems. It's the most important solution."

—John Mackey, vegan, founder and CEO, Whole Foods Market

"No one cares about your protein intake until they hear you're vegan!"

—Every single vegan

It's up to you. You're the one who lives in your body, wants a change, hopes for an answer, wishes for a miracle. Fortunately, you're holding one! It's the Clear Skin Diet, and you should be feeling excited, ready to go, brimming with enthusiasm to start putting your acne behind you. But maybe some of the people around you are skeptical. Maybe they're going to try to push you off your center, dent your enthusiasm, beat you down, shake your resolve. Maybe they'll say, "Oh come on, one bite of this cheesecake isn't going to cause your entire face to break out! Lighten up!"

Nope. Wrong. Don't lighten up. This is your face, your body, your health, your life. You have to decide to be the person who's going to make a difference for yourself and keep things positive. The Clear Skin Diet is how you need to be eating; don't let anyone tell you otherwise.

Put in the time and commitment to get the results you want because that's what you deserve. This lifestyle is the solution to a lot of major health problems, so dip into your emotional resolve and ignore the haters. After all, you've got nothing to lose except your acne.

But when your friends and family find out you've adopted a healthy plant-based diet, a funny thing might happen. Some of them may suddenly become "experts" in nutrition. Even though they've never mentioned the rampant obesity, heart disease, cancer, or type 2 diabetes associated with the standard American diet, heavy with meat, dairy, and processed food, they are supremely concerned that you are eating only fruits, vegetables, and whole grains. Apparently, they need to save you from your "unhealthy" or "downright dangerous" vegan diet because everyone knows that consuming plants instead of hot dogs is terrifying, right?

ACNE ADVICE:
From Neal Barnard, MD

If you live with others, ask for their support or invite them to join you! If people try to tease you, just tell them this is how you're eating right now and ask again for their support.

Understandably, friends and family may have questions or even concerns if you're trying something unfamiliar to them. And let's face it: there's a lot of conflicting information about nutrition, and most people really don't have a clue what healthy nutrition is. Why is that? The unfortunate fact is a lot of nutritional information we're exposed to these days, including government dietary recommendations, are twisted to benefit the food industry.

DOCTORS ONCE RECOMMENDED SMOKING CIGARETTES

To understand why you can't trust a lot of nutrition research today, we're going to look back to 1964 when the *Report of the Surgeon General's Advisory Committee on Smoking and Health* was published. This report had a devastating impact on the tobacco industry. Authored by then-surgeon general Luther Terry, MD, it was the first report linking smoking to lung cancer. Before that, most experts believed that smoking was good for you, and doctors even appeared in cigarette advertisements. This 1964 report documented unequivocally how smoking caused cancer and was extremely dangerous to your health.

Right after the press conference announcing this report, Dr. Terry was asked by a reporter whether he himself smoked. "No sir," Dr. Terry replied. "I don't."

"Dr. Terry, have you ever smoked?"

"Yes, I used to," he said.

"Dr. Terry, when did you quit?"

"Ten minutes ago."[1]

In 1964, when the report was released, 50 percent of US adults smoked. And it wasn't just bars that were filled with clouds of cigarette smoke. You couldn't walk into a restaurant, movie theater, store, or even doctor's office without getting hit by the smell of tobacco. People used to smoke in hospitals! It seems weird now, but smoking just a few decades ago was a huge health problem. Since the 1964 report's publication, the percentage of smokers in the US population has steadily decreased, from 50 percent to about 17 percent of the adult population today. Smoking is now banned in many public places. The report's publication is seen as a major turning point in public acceptance of the dangers of smoking and a crushing economic blow to the tobacco business.

MEAT AND DAIRY INDUSTRIES DON'T WANT TO END UP LIKE TOBACCO

In 1977 the government produced another important public health report—but this time about food. Called the McGovern Report, it was the product of the bipartisan Senate Select Committee on Human and Nutrition Needs, and the report's initial draft contained very strong conclusions about food choices and their relationship to disease. It advised that the public should eat "less meat, less fat, less saturated fat, less cholesterol...and more fruits, vegetables and cereal products." The McGovern Report promoted an increase in the intake of starches—whole grains, legumes and root vegetables, green and yellow nonstarchy vegetables, and fruits. Based on solid scientific research, the report recommended that meat, milk, butter, cheese, salt, and simple sugars should all be reduced in order to promote better health.

When the McGovern Report was initially published, the food industry went ballistic. The meat and dairy industries weren't going to let a government health report do to their sales what the surgeon general's report on smoking did to tobacco. The animal food industry did everything in its power to downplay the 1977 McGovern Report. The meat and dairy industries hired lobbyists, paid medical and nutrition experts to provide meat-friendly opinions, made campaign donations to politicians, and bought huge positive ad campaigns for their products. They were successful at having the recommendations in the McGovern Report highly watered down before it was publicly released. Mentions of specific foods, like meat, milk, eggs, and cheese were removed from the report. The report only used code words like *saturated fat, cholesterol,* or *excess protein.* Rather than be direct and tell people specifically which foods are healthiest and which should be avoided or limited, these more vague terms were used—in a nod to the animal food industries.

In the early 1980s the animal food industries began aggressively funding nutrition research that favored their own products in order to promote sales and create marketing hype. This is the primary reason so much contradictory nutrition information appears today in the scientific literature. Industry control over science is a very serious and significant issue. In fact, Marcia Angell, MD, who for the past twenty years has been editor in chief of the *New England Journal of Medicine*—one of the most respected medical journals on earth—recently wrote: "It is simply no longer possible to believe much of the clinical research that is published, or to rely on the judgment of trusted physicians or authoritative medical guidelines. I take no pleasure in this conclusion, which I reached slowly and reluctantly over my two decades as an editor of *The New England Journal of Medicine*."

While Dr. Angell largely decries drug research paid for and controlled by Big Pharma, the same holds true for Big Food. Most nutrition research published in the past thirty-five years was paid for by the companies selling the very food being studied. Positive-sounding research about milk? Paid for by the dairy industry. Research suggesting meat is essential? Paid for by the meat industry. Research saying eat nuts or die sooner? Paid for by the nut industry. How often do you think an industry has willingly funded a study that proves its product is bad? Practically never. And when it does, the industry can often prevent the study results from being published.

Marion Nestle, PhD, MPH, the Paulette Goddard Professor of Nutrition, Food Studies, and Public Health at New York University, examined this problem in detail. Professor Nestle spent a year tracking industry-funded studies on food. Her conclusion? "Roughly 90 percent of nearly 170 studies *favored the sponsor's interest,*" she discovered. We've all heard of fake news? Fake science has been around for a while now, too, because the food industry regularly finances very weak or even misleading research, with the hope of increasing sales of their products.

MOST DOCTORS HAVE LITTLE NUTRITIONAL KNOWLEDGE

Another obstacle to getting accurate information about nutrition is that most doctors aren't educated about how food impacts your body. Medical students receive fewer than twenty hours of nutrition education during four years of medical school. Nutrition professionals who've studied this say it is completely "inadequate."[2]

It's well established in modern scientific literature that heart disease, type 2 diabetes, autoimmune diseases, and even many forms of cancer can be prevented and often reversed through a healthy, low-fat, plant-based diet. Yet many doctors are completely unaware of this science, or too busy to look for alternatives to drugs, or pressured by patients to find a quick fix. They continue to prescribe medications and procedures that treat symptoms but don't actually address the underlying problem. It's worth noting that nutrition studies that show a healthy plant-based diet can arrest and reverse many serious diseases are not being funded by big business. This is because there is nothing to "sell" from research showing, for instance, that you can 100 percent cure heart disease by just eating potatoes, beans, and veggies. Thus, there is no marketing or PR budget to get this information out widely to doctors or the public. Contrast that with research about drugs, and you understand why there are expensive PR campaigns and continuous high-budget TV commercials every five minutes for the latest pill. Unless you pick up a book like this one, most people won't get to learn about the power of plant-only diets.

This is the background for what you might be contending with when your friends find out you only eat plants, and then become hyperconcerned about your well-being.

ACNE ADVICE:
From Ann Esselstyn

You may feel alone or frustrated that the people you care about aren't with you in your plant-based journey, but have confidence that you are sending a strong message of the power of whole food and plant-based nutrition, and people you would never imagine are listening and looking!

THE BENEFITS OF LOW-FAT PLANT-BASED DIETS ARE ENORMOUS

Despite the power and money wielded by the animal food industries, a plant-only diet is steadily gaining traction. More and more people are discovering its numerous health benefits. One of the nation's largest health plans, the Kaiser Permanente Medical Group, produced a very useful document called "Nutritional Update for Physicians: Plant-Based Diets."[3] It appeared in a peer-reviewed journal with the scientific references to back everything up. The paper summarized research on plant-only diets.

Citing detailed, published, solid research, the Kaiser Permanente review focused on five proven benefits of plant-only diets:

1. Plant-based diets prevent and reverse obesity and should be encouraged for all ages.
2. Plant-based diets can prevent and reverse type 2 diabetes.
3. Plant-based diets lower high blood pressure.
4. Plant-based diets can prevent and reverse heart disease, America's number-one killer.
5. Plant-based diets can reduce mortality compared with non-plant-based diets. Patients can live longer and have less cancer if they go plant-based.

The Kaiser Permanente update is packed with numerous cites from scientific literature underscoring the health benefits of plant-only diets.[4] Imagine if a drug company came up with a pill that would make you lose excess weight, no longer require medications you may be taking, and dramatically decrease your risk of cancer and heart disease. That drug company would make a fortune because everyone would want that pill! But you can get *all* those benefits and more, just by eating the Clear Skin Diet. If you weren't already excited, you should be now.

EXPLODING SOME MYTHS

What should you do if someone you care about starts warning you that your new plant-only diet may be unhealthy? We've put together questions we have heard in one form or another, basically our whole lives, with answers for your curious friends and family members. Sometimes you may get questions that

ACNE ADVICE:
From Jeff Novick, MS, RD

Realize that in today's environment, everyone has become an "expert" on diet and health, and so people are often asking about your diet because they want to challenge or debate you. They may want to defend their own habits or information they are following. I don't engage in these debates or challenges and don't recommend you do either. You just end up exhausted, stressed, and irritated, and that is not a good way to live. So, do this diet for yourself, stay focused, avoid the latest health hype and trends, and stay on the path of enjoying good, healthful foods and all the benefits. If someone notices and wants to learn more, share information and resources. If they disagree, that's fine. Just keep taking care of you, your skin, and your overall health.

are sort of antagonistic and more about the other person's discomfort at your new diet than actual interest in your health. In those cases, it might be best just to answer by saying, "You may be right, I'm not sure. But the diet seems to be working pretty well for me right now, so I'm going to keep with it." It's hard to argue with an answer like that and usually ends the interrogation. But if you want to arm yourself with facts, here are some common questions and answers:

1. WILL I NEED TO TAKE A B12 SUPPLEMENT?

Vitamin B12 is a nutrient that helps keep the body's nerve and blood cells healthy and helps make DNA, the genetic material in all cells. Vitamin B12 also helps prevent a type of anemia called megaloblastic anemia, which makes people tired and weak. People going on a 100 percent plant-based diet over the long term will want to supplement vitamin B12 at some point. Vitamin B12 is found in plentiful supply in nature, such as in dirt. When animals eat plants, they eat a small amount of dirt on the plant and absorb some B12—enough for their small requirements. If you eat that animal, you can then absorb some of that B12, which was stored in the animal's tissue, and that way you get the small amount of B12 you require. Because modern food farming and preparation emphasizes thoroughly cleaning and washing fruits and veggies, there is very little dirt on the plant foods you buy at the supermarket, meaning there will be very little, if any, B12 on them. This is why people who eat a plant-based diet need to take B12.

B12 is stored in your liver, and most people will have an adequate supply for two to five years from the time they stop eating animal products to when they may require supplementation. We encourage people to follow Dr. McDougall's guidelines and begin taking a vitamin B12 supplement. We recommend you wait to start that B12 until after your acne has cleared, or up to two years. Research suggests a small percentage of people may be susceptible to acne outbreaks triggered by high doses of B12, like the dose levels found in commercial B12 supplements. This is why you should not begin B12 supplementation right away. We cover this in more detail in chapter 6.

2. WILL I GET ENOUGH PROTEIN?

We guarantee you'll get this question at least once a day. And the good news is, you will get plenty of protein on the Clear Skin Diet. Most Americans are actually getting way too much protein. Most people associate the benefits of lots of protein with words like *muscle, vitality, strength, power, energy, aggressiveness,* and *liveliness.* In fact, more accurate words would be *bone loss, osteoporosis, kidney damage, kidney stones, arthritis, cancer promotion, low energy,* and *overall poor health.* These are all consequences from overloading protein in your diet. Some protein is good, but more is not better. Taking in excess protein is a hazard to

ACNE ADVICE:
From John McDougall, MD

A protein deficient diet is impossible! Protein is so abundant in plant foods that it is impossible to design a diet based on starches and vegetables that fails to provide for the needs of children and adults. Experimental studies carried out in the 1940s and 1950s showed that people require about 2.5 percent of their calories as protein. In order to provide a definitely safe level—to cover situations such as chronic infection and injuries—the World Health Organization (WHO) doubled these figures. Since 1974, WHO has recommended that men, women, and children consume about 5 percent of their calories as protein. Pregnant women should consume about 6.5 percent of their calories as protein, and lactating women 7 percent.

No one would contest that the ideal food for a baby is human breast milk, which is only 5 percent protein. Commonly consumed starches and vegetables contain from 6 to 45 percent of their calories as protein and therefore are more than sufficient to supply the protein needs of children and adults, who grow at a much slower rate than babies.

your health, just like taking in excess cholesterol or fat. Excess protein is actually a known problem reported on by scientists for more than a century. People have little awareness of protein overload, however. Any more than 10 percent of calories from protein is likely excessive and can promote the chronic diseases mentioned above, especially when the protein is from an animal source. Unlike fat or carbohydrates, both of which your body can store if you overconsume it, excess protein cannot be stored. And due to its acid nature, protein has to be buffered in order to prevent your body's pH level from becoming too acidic. To do that, the body leeches calcium from your bones and neutralizes the acid load. Over time, leeching calcium to neutralize excess acidic protein load can promote a number of problems, such as osteoporosis (thinning of the bones).

How often have you heard of someone being hospitalized for protein deficiency? Never. If you're eating enough calories, you will get an adequate amount of protein. Protein deficiency is only recorded in the scientific literature when someone is starving to death. In that case, the problem is not actually protein deficiency, but overall calorie deficiency.

Top medical doctors like John McDougall, Neal Barnard, Dean Ornish, Caldwell Esselstyn, Leila Masson, and Irminne Van Dyken, agree that the naturally occurring amount of protein in a healthy plant-based diet is more than adequate. By following the Clear Skin Diet, you're going to be getting the optimal amount of protein and avoiding the health challenges brought on by excess animal protein intake. So there.

3. WILL I GET ENOUGH CALCIUM?

And the other half of that question typically includes, "Don't you need milk (from a cow) for calcium?" Here's your answer. A varied plant-only diet offers some of the best calcium sources available. Best yet, you can escape the damaging health effects associated with dairy products (e.g., acne).

Good plant sources of calcium include all green leafy vegetables, oranges, kidney beans, lima beans, whole grains, lentils, raisins, broccoli, kale, celery, and romaine lettuce (acne-busting foods!).

Many people mistakenly believe that they need to ingest high levels of calcium in order to stave off osteoporosis (weakening of the bones). We've been brainwashed from a young age to believe this, thanks to propaganda from the dairy industry.

In fact, there is no calcium deficiency that causes or contributes to osteoporosis. Studies show that countries with the highest rate of dairy intake, like the United States, New Zealand, Britain, and Sweden, also have the highest incidence of osteoporosis. One reason people in these countries have such high levels of the disease is because of their excessive consumption of animal protein, which leaches calcium from their bones. It's not a lack of calcium consumption causing problems. It is excessive protein, coupled with a lack of exercise, that's causing osteoporosis. In other words, milk is harmful, not beneficial.

Our hero, John McDougall, MD, has written extensively about the research surrounding calcium and dairy intake. Countries with very low dairy consumption, like China, have almost no cases of osteoporosis. Consider this: even dairy-industry-funded research shows that dairy doesn't fight osteoporosis. One study funded by the National Dairy Council looked at the effects of fluid milk on postmenopausal women. The study showed participants who received extra milk (three eight-ounce glasses of skimmed milk daily) for a year lost more bone than those who didn't drink the extra milk.[5] The study authors, Recker and Heaney, wrote, "The protein content of the milk supplement may have a negative effect on calcium balance, possibly through an increase in kidney losses of calcium or through a direct effect on bone resorption...this may have been due to the average 30 percent increase in protein intake during milk supplementation." The dairy industry itself is fully aware that milk does not build strong bones but actually *harms* bones. Avoiding animal protein—including dairy products—is the best thing you can do for your bones. No milk for you!

4. WON'T CARBS MAKE ME FAT?

This one kind of cracks us up. The simple answer is *no*. We are lifelong athletes who fuel our activities with carbs. We've never had weight issues. When someone says something like this to you, remember they are just caring, curious, or both.

The fact is not all carbs are created equal. Sugar is a carb; so are carrots and apples. Sugar mixed with fat can promote weight gain, because sugar raises insulin to help drive the fat into your fat cells. But carbs have gotten an undeserved negative rap in the press. Whole food carbs like starches are not fattening foods because the body has to work hard to convert complex carbohydrates into fat. Sugar alone doesn't necessarily contribute much fat either. In fact, scientists agree that starch and sugar *are not* easily converted into fat, and their conclusions are solidly backed up in the scientific literature.[6]

Carbohydrates consumed in excess of what we need are usually burned off as heat or used in physical movements beyond exercise (called fidgeting movements). Humans are inefficient at turning carbohydrates into fat, a process known as de novo lipogenesis. Humans expend 30 percent of the excess carbohydrate calories just in the process of converting them to fat, which is a wasteful process.[7]

There is a body of research testing de novo lipogenesis in humans. In these studies, researchers gave large amounts of excess sugars to subjects, and then documented that the subjects only gained a small amount of fat, rather than what might have been expected from the excess sugar calories. In one study, for example, women were given 50 percent more calories than they usually ate in a day, along with another 3.5 ounces (or almost 400 calories) of refined sugar. At the end of thirty days eating all these extra calories plus nearly 12,000 extra calories of sugar every day, the women had only gained one extra pound of body fat (which represents 3,500 calories).[8] This can help explain why people who eat diets high in carbohydrates like rice—in Asia, for example—tend to be thinner than Americans and Europeans, who consume diets high in animal products and tend to be overweight or obese.

The Clear Skin Diet will not make you gain weight. The Clear Skin Diet will help you maintain or achieve your optimal weight.

5. WILL I GET ENOUGH ESSENTIAL FATS? DO I NEED ANY SUPPLEMENTS?

Here's the deal. A whole food starch-based diet provides all your nutrient and fat requirements in the ideal amounts and in the ideal packaging. Fruits, vegetables, and other plant foods have everything you need.

Your body can synthesize nearly all of the organic compounds required to build and maintain itself. There are a handful of elements it can't synthesize and that need to come from food. In total, eleven vitamins, eight amino acids, and two kinds of fat must come from food. All of these essential nutrients are made by plants and are found in abundant supply in the Clear Skin Diet (the only exceptions are vitamin D, which comes from sun exposure, and B12, which comes from bacteria). Omega-3 and omega-6 fats (called essential fats) are only made by plants, and you easily get them by eating plant foods (or by eating animals that have gotten them from plants themselves).

Essential fats play an important role in our bodies to make cells and hormones. Our requirement for essential fats is tiny, and even the most basic natural diets supply sufficient linoleic acid to meet our requirement. This is why, in practical terms, a condition of essential fatty acid deficiency just does not happen in populations eating fruits and vegetables and is of zero concern when eating a healthy, low-fat, plant-based diet. Other than B12, no supplements are necessary on the Clear Skin Diet. Some physicians do recommend zinc for acne sufferers, but that's entirely optional.

6. ISN'T THIS DIET BORING?

I guess if you're used to eating pastries, cookies, burgers, cheesy pizzas—that is, the diet many Americans devour—eating a healthy diet instead may, at first, seem slightly less thrilling. Drive-through food—oily, salty, sugary, high calorie—is a much bigger dopamine brain charge than healthy food. If your eating style prior to the Clear Skin Diet has been high-calorie, super-stimulating, unhealthy foods, you may find that it takes a slightly longer period of time before your palate changes and healthy food starts tasting as delicious as it is.

Eating a simple, healthy, starch-based diet can be a joyful experience. Over the first weeks your taste buds will begin to adjust, and you will start to discover how food tastes when it isn't disguised in oil. Oily, goopy sauces hide the true flavor of many dishes. Foods actually taste better and more real when you take out the butter, margarine, or sour cream. Each plant has a unique taste, and your palate will appreciate and want those special flavors.

ACNE ADVICE:
From Chef AJ

It's not always even necessary to tell people about your diet unless they are genuinely interested and ask. But I believe that a picture is worth a thousand words, so why not carry a before and after photo on your phone, and when they ask why you eat this way, you can show them how successful you have been with your new diet!

7. DON'T I NEED ANIMAL PROTEIN TO BE AN ACTIVE ATHLETE?

More and more athletes—professional and amateur—are adopting plant-only diets, and in the process they not only get healthier but deliver some of their best athletic performances. Ultramarathon runner Scott Jurek, MMA champion Mac Danzig, Olympic athlete Meryeta O'Dine (snowboarder), NFL Linebacker David Carter (aka "The 300 Pound Vegan"), power-lifter Alison Crowdus, Portland Trail Blazers' Damian Lillard, Denver Nuggets forward Wilson Chandler, Formula One racer Lewis Hamilton, tennis champion Venus Williams, bodybuilder Jehina Malik, professional surfer Tia Blanco—these are just a few of the scores of plant-powered professional athletes who dominate their sports, and the list is growing daily.

If you're an athlete, adopting the Clear Skin Diet could make your own athletic performance improve markedly.

8. SHOULD I EAT TEN BANANAS FOR BREAKFAST AND TWENTY ORANGES FOR LUNCH?

No. If you've spent time on the Internet you may have seen a variety of odd vegan diets. They're marketed by passionate individuals who swear by them and may promote them with bikini or fitness photos. These diets may be healthier than the standard diet most Americans eat, and everyone can certainly eat any diet they wish, but just know that these diets—whether a raw diet, or raw-until-whenever diet, or a high olive oil diet—are not diets based on any sound science. They are "guru-based" diets where you have to accept on faith that the diets do what the guru marketing them claims they do. (They generally don't.) The Clear Skin Diet is based on actual, solid, peer-reviewed, and published research and is used in clinical settings by many top physicians and dietitians. It's the same diet pattern consumed for many generations by the longest-lived, healthiest cultures ever studied. If you want to heal your acne, starches and veggies are what you need, not a super fruit-heavy diet, which can be inconvenient, hard to maintain, less satiating, actually problematic over the long term for your health—and may not resolve acne for some people.

—◇—

DIET STOPS ACNE: ROBYN FERRIS, AGE 25

Robyn lives in England and saw a YouTube video we made announcing our second Acne Intervention Program, which we presented through the Internet. Robyn contacted us and said she had had hormonal acne on her chin, jaw, and neck for twelve years. She'd tried many different approaches to get it under control, like antibiotics and topical treatments. Sometimes the medications worked and reduced her acne. But once she stopped taking them, the acne always returned, much to Robyn's frustration.

Robyn said that it took a "solid two months" for her to begin seeing some really great improvements. Her problem chin area and her overall skin quality was smoother and better. Robyn has some expected post-inflammatory hyper-pigmentation (PIH), the flat spots of slightly darker skin tone that can some-times linger after acne has stopped. PIH can takes a little more time to fade once your acne's stopped—but these areas *do* fade (see chapter 8).

Everyone is different in terms of how long the Clear Skin Diet takes to bring about impressive results. For Robyn, it took months, but she showed that great results come to those who persevere.

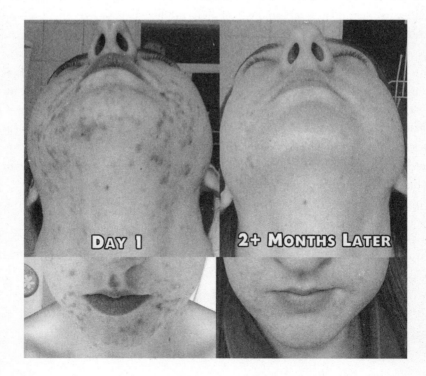

6

THE ELIMINATION DIET AND OTHER TROUBLESHOOTING STRATEGIES

by Nina

"The elimination diet: Remove anger, regret, resentment, guilt, blame, and worry. Then watch your health, and life, improve."

—Dr. Charles Glassman, MD

"Success is the sum of small efforts repeated day in and day out."

—Unknown

The Clear Skin Diet is designed as a six-week program. We selected that time frame because our Acne Intervention Programs showed that this was the average time most people required to experience sufficient improvement in their skin. Some participants required eight weeks or more to begin seeing their desired results; others only needed two. Everyone loves instant gratification. However, the reality is, solid success often takes more time, effort, and tweaking for some people. But even if it takes five or six months on the Clear Skin Diet to be rid of acne, keeping to this diet is well worth it. Five or six months is much faster than never. Be patient!

When someone tells me he or she has tried the Clear Skin Diet but couldn't get it to work, I want to ask: Did you actually follow the diet 100 percent? Usually the person hasn't. Real change won't happen if you are still eating the occasional added fats like nuts, seeds, avocados, olives, soybeans, coconuts, or oil.

Cheryl was a fifteen-year-old participant in our first intervention group. She had pretty severe acne and initially found us by doing a search on YouTube about acne cures. She was hoping that being part of our acne intervention group would give her the support and education she needed to succeed. Cheryl shared how she had actually attempted to do our Clear Skin Diet program on her own, but it hadn't worked for her. As we talked through her experience, Cheryl conceded that she had been doing the diet "maybe 90 or 95 percent." She told us her family was eating out at a local vegan restaurant a few times a month. There wasn't anything compliant available, so she was stuck with ordering fatty vegan treat food. It's delicious but can wreak havoc on sensitive skin.

Ninety or 95 percent isn't doing the program; 100 percent is doing the program. You have to think of your body as being food sensitive. For some people, even a small indiscretion can show up as a breakout within a day. Eating an oily veggie burger one night because there was nothing else on the menu—that's not doing the program. People in acne-free cultures don't take a night off every so often and have something greasy or oily. Consistency is your friend. Cheryl resolved to do the program 100 percent, and at the end of thirty days of being strict, she was making good progress in stopping her acne.

Another of our Acne Intervention Program participants, Carmen from Mexico City, initially cleared a lot of her acne very quickly. But about a month into the program, she reported feeling the diet had made her more sensitive to fats because she said that even just a small slip resulted in a breakout. Eating even just a small amount of a fatty food was causing Carmen's pimples to return, she complained. In fact, the Clear Skin Diet was working for Carmen, and the proof was that when she deviated from the diet, her acne came back. The message to Carmen was simple: try to do better avoiding the foods you now realize cause your acne. If you don't slip, you won't have acne.

If you're not seeing the results you want yet, review your food log and examine what you have been eating closely. If you have not kept a record of your food intake, start now. Are you really doing the program 100 percent? One hundred percent compliance is the price for becoming acne-free, at least in the beginning, while you are starting to contain breakouts.

It may take more time for those on the more severe end of the spectrum to achieve those startling before and after pictures. Your skin will progress through various phases as it heals. Your acne can be clearing as it should be, but you may have Post Inflammatory Pigmentation (red spots), or you may have scarring.

Both can be treated with dermatological tools (which we discuss more in depth in chapter 8). Be confident that you are making progress by reducing active acne, even if there is still damage, artifacts, or scarring yet to be dealt with later.

STRATEGIES FOR STUBBORN SKIN

Based on our acne intervention pilot studies, many people will get very fast results and see their acne begin clearing up within a few weeks. For others, it will take longer before fading begins. This is not unusual when dealing with serious skin conditions. Dermatologists advise that Accutane can take more than four months to begin working on some patients, if it even does. So don't obsess if you're one of those people who does not see immediate results. Nearly every compliant participant in our study groups experienced marked improvement within eight to twelve weeks of starting the diet.

ACNE ADVICE:
From Irminne Van Dyken, MD

Let me introduce you to the gut microbiome—a fascinating collection of microbes including bacteria, viruses, and fungi that live on and within our bodies. These microbes outnumber us ten to one, meaning for every one of our human cells there are ten microbial cells that live on and within us. This translates to two to five pounds of our overall body weight being microbes! They influence our overall health—and our skin—more than we ever could have imagined. Only recently have we discovered a connection between the microbiome and acne. Scientists have called it the gut-brain-skin connection, and they have demonstrated that we can manipulate this connection to our advantage.

When your bacterial balance is off, and there are more unhealthy than healthy bacteria, it is called dysbiosis. In dysbiosis unhealthy bacterial populations break down the protective layer of your intestines and contribute to a condition called leaky gut. When this happens, the tight junctions between the one-cell-layer-thick gut lining that are leak proof spread farther apart, allowing inflammatory chemicals and toxins to leave the gut, enter the body, and wreak havoc.

Acne is an inflammatory disease, and scientists have measured an increase in inflammatory mediators in people with acne. Eating healthy leads to a healthy gut microbiome. This, in turn, leads to decreased inflammation in the body and decreased leaky gut. Decreased leaky gut in turn leads to decreased acne formation.

(continues)

Irminne Van Dyken, MD *(continued)*

So how can we eat for a healthy microbiome?

Prebiotics. Prebiotics are certain foods that contain nondigestible fiber compounds, but once they reach our colon, our bacteria there consumes them. Eating prebiotics feeds the healthy bacteria in our intestines. Examples of prebiotic foods are garlic, onions, jicama, dandelion greens, chicory, and Jerusalem artichokes.

Fiber. Not all foods with fiber are prebiotics. Soluble fiber also supports the microbiome by providing the optimal intestinal environment for healthy bacterial growth. Try to get a minimum of forty grams of overall fiber in your diet daily. A high-fiber diet has also been shown to improve acne.

Probiotics. Probiotics are live microorganisms that can be added to your diet. Adding them to the regimen will improve the diversity of your gut microbiome and lead to healthier bacterial populations. Probiotics can be found in fermented foods such as kombucha, kimchi, miso, tempeh, and sauerkraut. It may even be useful to take a probiotic supplement initially to jump-start your healthy bacterial populations. Just make sure your probiotic is a quality one, with over fifty billion colony-forming units (CFU) and at least five different bacterial strains. Specific to acne, multiple scientific studies have demonstrated that taking a probiotic supplement daily decreases the length and severity of acne breakouts. Scientists speculate this is due to reduced systemic inflammation and oxidative stress as prebiotic supplementation has been shown to reduce these.

Avoid antibiotics. Of course, there is no doubt that antibiotics save countless lives. There are instances when they are necessary, but there are many more instances where they are unnecessarily prescribed. One course of broad spectrum antibiotics (for example something given for a cold) can kill off one-third of the microbiome. After devastation like that, it is hard work to rebuild microbial diversity and regain a healthy microbe balance. As a rule, if your doctor wants to prescribe antibiotics, ask yourself and the doctor, are they really necessary? If the answer is no, don't take them.

For more on prebiotics and acne, see "Edible Plants and Their Influence on the Gut Microbiome and Acne."[1]

GLUTEN AND B12

If you have followed the Clear Skin Diet conscientiously for three or more months and aren't improving, don't be discouraged. If you still have some new breakouts, you may have a sensitivity to a particular food or foods that are permitted on the Clear Skin Diet. Gluten is a common trigger, and it's possible you have gluten sensitivity. You may want to go gluten-free. If after a couple of months of adhering strictly to the Clear Skin Diet (especially when dining out), you're still experiencing breakouts, consider eliminating gluten. Examine your skin after two or three weeks without gluten, and if your acne has calmed down significantly, then you know you're onto something.

As mentioned in the last chapter, we do not recommend you start a vitamin B12 supplement right away, but only after you have cleared your acne completely or after two years of being vegan. Vitamin B12 is stored in your liver and most people will have an adequate supply for two to five years from the time they stop eating animal products. There are also vegan foods that add B12 supplementation. If you are already taking B12 and your acne is not clearing, we suggest you stop altogether for at least three months. Research has shown that high-dose B12 supplements may cause acne in a small percentage of people. It's relatively rare, but some people may be susceptible to this. This might be because an excess of B12 can alter the *P. acnes* bacteria on your skin in a way that promotes an inflammatory response, leading to new breakouts.

The average female adult requires 2.4 to 2.8 mcg of B12 per day, but when you look at the labels of commonly available B12 supplements, they can be 1,000 to 2,000 mcg per dose. High amounts of B12 are considered safe because it is a water-soluble vitamin and your body will excrete any excess through your urine.

ACNE ADVICE:
From Leila Masson, MD

When I see young people with acne I often think of zinc. Zinc is a mineral needed to fight bacteria and infections, reduce inflammation, and heal skin—and all these processes are involved in acne. Humans need more zinc when they grow fast, such as in adolescence. Therefore the daily requirement for a teenager may be higher than that of an adult, and it may be difficult to meet this requirement with diet alone. We used to get our zinc from eating vegetables and legumes grown in healthy soil; but nowadays because of intensive farming practices, many soils are overfarmed and depleted of zinc. Low zinc levels in the body can promote acne, stretch marks, recurrent infections, and low moods. I have seen many teenagers become happier and healthier once their zinc deficiency was treated properly: their frustration tolerance improved significantly and their acne-prone skin healed—to the delight of their parents and themselves! You can get a blood test to check for plasma zinc, and if it is low, your health provider can recommend the right dose for you.

The four main B12 supplements available are hydroxocobalamin, cyanoco-balamin, methylcobalamin, and adenosylcobalamin. If you quit B12 and your acne stops, you can later experiment with different types of B12, in the lowest reasonable dose, and see if you break out on the other varieties. But again, breakouts from B12 sensitivity are thought to affect a very small percentage of people.

ELIMINATION DIET

The elimination diet is for people who follow the Clear Skin Diet for three or four months and, despite doing everything right, still experience some breakouts. Elimination diets have been around for a long time and are a tool used by doctors to identify food sensitivities and allergies. People with autoimmune diseases, leaky gut syndrome, and other allergies have used elimination diets to identify the specific foods contributing to their problems. Our elimination diet is based on diets used by Dr. John McDougall, Dr. Michael Klaper, and Dr. Neal Barnard. You can find each of their elimination diets on their websites (see Resources).

With the elimination diet, you are going to follow a very neutral, plain, basic diet that should calm your acne completely. Then you will add back foods one at a time and watch to see if you start breaking out. In this way, you can find out which foods you need to avoid.

Before you institute the elimination diet, please be sure you have already ruled out other possible triggers discussed in this book, such as vitamin B12, skin care and makeup products, laundry detergents (described ahead in chapter 7). If you've eliminated those as possible influences and been 100 percent compliant on the Clear Skin Diet for at least three months—and are still experiencing new breakouts—you're a candidate for the elimination diet.

ELIMINATION DIET GUIDELINES

1. Eliminate soy foods. The elimination diet excludes processed foods, fake foods, so no soy, including fat-free soymilks.
2. Go gluten-free (no wheat, barley, or rye). These items can be found in cereals, pastas, and breads. A certain percentage of people have been found to react to gluten, including having adverse skin reactions.

3. Avoid all citrus fruits such as oranges, lemons, limes, and grape-fruits; also no apples, bananas, peaches, or tomatoes

4. Eat 80 percent starches and 20 percent cooked vegetables and cooked fruits. Cook all foods completely before eating, including fruits. Boiling and steaming are the healthiest ways to do this, but microwaving is acceptable. You are not going to be eating any raw or uncooked foods on the elimination diet. Cooking alters the proteins in foods, making them less likely to provoke allergic responses.

5. Here are the foods you should consume:
   - ❖ Rice, especially brown rice.
   - ❖ Cooked green vegetables, such as broccoli, spinach, Swiss chard, lettuce, collards, string beans, asparagus, spinach.
   - ❖ Cooked yellow and orange vegetables, such as carrots or sweet potatoes, beets, beet greens, chard, artichokes, celery, summer squash.
   - ❖ Cooked *noncitrus* fruits, such as apricots, berries, cherries, cranberries, papaya, plums, prunes.
   - ❖ Drink only plain water or carbonated water, such as Perrier. Avoid all other beverages, including coffee and teas of any kind. We want to err on the side of caution.
   - ❖ Salt is the only condiment allowed—this means no salad dress-ings, lemon juice, mustard, vinegar, sugar, or other condiments. We want to prevent any allergic response and make the diet completely simple and basic.

The elimination diet goes nuclear on lingering acne. It will take at least a week after you have begun following the elimination diet for your intestines to clear, but it can take longer for your acne to calm. Once your acne has subsided, with no new breakouts, you can begin adding back the foods you eliminated. Add back only one new food at a time, though. This is the easiest way to determine whether or not that given food was the troublemaker. One of our Facebook group members cleared her acne completely with six weeks of the elimination diet. When she began adding back in foods, she discovered that oats, glutens, nightshades, and some fruits caused her acne to return.

In order to test a given new food, eat that new food three times a day, at every meal and in large amounts. Do this for three days, eating large amounts of the test food at each meal. If by the end of three days you are not noticing any breakout or other skin problems, you can conclude that this food is not a trigger food for your acne. You can then keep that new food in your diet going forward. Anything that causes acne through this testing should be eliminated. Once you are ready, move on to the next food in question. Don't add two new foods at the same time because if you experience a reaction, you won't know which food is the cause. Keep your diet simple throughout this process. Keep it consistent, so when you add a new food, you will be able to detect whether that food is an acne culprit for you.

Note that if you add a food back and get an acne reaction, you should drop that food right away. Continue on the elimination diet for a full week before adding any new food. A week without another new food gives you time to clear the trigger food from your system.

Remember that you are not experimenting with any foods that are prohibited in the diet. For example, you won't add in avocados, nuts, or oils to test at this point. You are only testing foods to find triggers that are part of the Clear Skin Diet. Once you have identified trigger foods, you can eat the full Clear Skin Diet for a few months (minus your trigger food) and continue healing your acne.

Here are foods you can add back to your elimination diet, once you are ready. Add them back in this order, beginning with the most gentle foods in the left column, followed by those in the right:

Bananas	Tomatoes
Apples	Wheat (bread, pasta, etc.)
Corn	Citrus fruits
Onions	Soy products

If there are any beverages you like, remember to add them separately and give each one three days to determine if it is a trigger.

Be sure to add foods back to your elimination diet in large amounts. A small amount may not trigger acne, whereas eating a larger amount of that new food over a few days could.

Be aware that women may have different kinds of triggers at different times of the month due to natural hormonal changes. If you identify foods that are only occasional triggers, you have learned to avoid those foods at certain times.

It is possible your triggers could change over time. If you go six months acne-free, and then suddenly acne begins showing up again, you may need to repeat the elimination diet to determine whether your sensitivities have changed.

If it ends up taking three, four, or even six months to identify triggers and eliminate your acne, you are way ahead. Doing nothing will only achieve nothing. We totally understand that you want your acne to disappear overnight, but please have the patience to wait 30 or 90 or 120 nights—the wait will have been worth it.

—◇—

DIET STOPS ACNE: KARA DELONAS, AGE 24

Kara started getting acne when she was eleven and struggled with it through-out her teenage years. The acne made her feel horrible. Kids bullied her, while nicer kids might say, "You'll be so pretty once your skin clears up!" Kara be-came adept at using makeup to hide her acne, but that didn't change the fact it was physically painful. She couldn't feel pretty without the makeup. Nothing the dermatologist gave Kara helped, and Proactiv made her skin so dry it actu-ally cracked in cold weather.

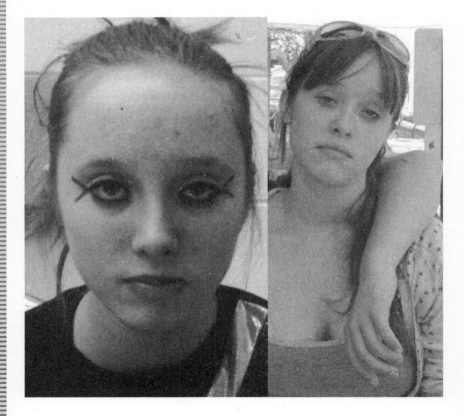

Kara said she was also insecure about her weight. As a triplet (two girls and a boy), Kara and her sister look a lot alike. Kids would comment about being able to tell them apart because Kara was heavier. This stung Kara, who later devel-oped bulimia, a serious eating disorder. Kara also had crippling migraines a few times a month, which usually lasted eight hours or more.

Kara discovered the Clear Skin Diet through the Internet: "Nina and Randa and their family put out videos and information that really helped teach how to eat in a healthy way. I actually started seeing results immediately. My acne became less intense at first, and then went away completely!"

Kara says she also lost weight and became more fit and felt stronger. Kara says she never purged again after going on this diet. "I don't weigh myself but think of myself as feeling stronger, as opposed to trying to be skinnier."

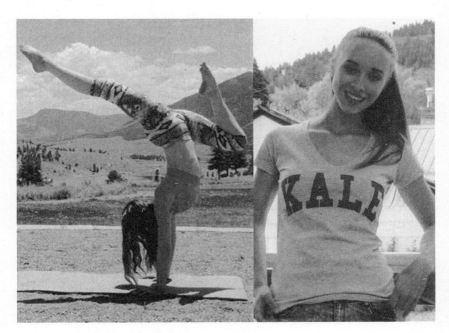

(See color photos in insert.)

PART II

COPING WITH ACNE

7

SKIN CARE IS SELF-CARE: YOUR CLEAR SKIN ENVIRONMENT

by Randa

"Self-care is never a selfish act—it is simply good stewardship of the only gift I have, the gift I was put on earth to offer to others."

—Parker Palmer

Do you know what the largest organ in your body is? Hint: It's not the brain, heart, or stomach. It's your skin! Your skin blankets your entire body, holding together the you that is you and covering more than three thousand square inches of your frame. Your skin protects you from impacts and pressure, notifies you of changes in temperature, and acts as a barrier. It regulates your body temperature and keeps your fluids in balance through sweat. Your skin senses heat, cold, touch, and pain with its massive network of nerve cells. The surface of your skin also reveals to others your vibrant good health, age, illness, and even your emotions.

One might think that something that plays such a vital role in our existence would be treated with respect, right? Wrong. People aren't necessarily all that kind to their skin. We bleach it, shave it, burn it, tattoo it, scrape it, scratch it, douse it in chemicals, and then wonder why our skin isn't in the kind of shape we'd like it to be.

Your skin just wants to be loved. Just imagine for a sec the big job it does for you day in and day out. Thank you, skin! As difficult as it might be when you are in the throes of any kind of acne breakout, you do need to learn to love your skin again. And part of that self-love means creating an environment in which your skin can thrive.

According to the research we've examined, it's apparent that acne is heavily influenced by environment. Your diet is the number one way you interact with your environment—you are literally ingesting your environment three times a day in the form of breakfast, lunch, and dinner. But while your diet may be the most important contributor to the clear skin environment, it's not the only one.

The people living in the acne-free zones are thriving in atmospheres that are probably far cleaner and less polluted than where you and I live. They are not using chemically processed personal care products on their faces and bodies—nor on their clothes, sheets, or towels either. We may not be lucky enough to live on pristine unpolluted islands, but we can certainly learn a lot from the people who do.

We can definitely replicate the diet of the people in the acne-free zones where those lucky young people not only have no acne but also avoid the emotional and physical stress provoked by bad skin. You can be that lucky too, but it's going to take some effort on your part. One of your most important tasks is to rethink the way you care for your skin.

ACNE ADVICE:
From Julieanna Hever, MS, RD

Ultimately, a healthful diet is the cornerstone for healthful skin—centering your meals on whole plant foods, abundant with leafy greens and carotenoid-rich red, orange, and yellow fruits and vegetables and drinking plenty of water throughout the day. But caring for your skin from the outside may help, too. Together, these habits will not only bring about immediately apparent results—clear, glowing skin—but will also pay dividends in your long-term health and beauty.

CLEAR SKIN GUIDELINES

The following are ten important clear skin guidelines to consider, regarding what you put on or against your skin. We're going to recommend some specific products and types of products, and you can refer to Appendix A: Recommended Products at the end of the book for a full list.

1. USE GENTLE, OIL-FREE PRODUCTS ONLY

People tend to use gallons of personal care products to try to cleanse their skin and hair. More is better, right? They are at war with their acne and always attacking it with the latest in blemish-fighting merchandise. Or perhaps they start washing their hair daily to get rid of the oil (even though daily washing actually makes hair produce *more* oil). Maybe you're using powders, foundations, concealers, and so on to hide a breakout (and that's OK, whatever it takes to get you through the day). But smothering your skin and hair with topicals can have a profound impact on your skin, and it's not always good. Some even actively promote acne, unfortunately.

The first rule in clear skin care is the same as diet—no oil! When you have acne-prone skin, you want to try avoid anything that contributes to the body's oil (sebum), which can clog your pores. Learn to become as diligent reading the ingredients of your personal care products as you are with your food. Make sure there is no oil in any of your skin-care or makeup products, including "essential oils." This includes your moisturizer, liquid foundation, powder, blush, makeup cleansing wipes, soap, sunscreen—basically anything that might go on your face. Your shampoos and conditioners can also come in contact with your face, so they need to be oil-free as well.

You might be doing the Clear Skin Diet perfectly, but your cleanser, makeup, or other skin-care products could be inhibiting your progress. What goes *on* your body is just as important as what goes in it. Don't touch your face any more than you have to, and when you do, make sure your hands are clean. You don't want to transfer anything oily from your hands to your face.

The following is a list of comedogenic (pore-clogging) ingredients to watch out for. Avoid buying products that contain these ingredients—and the fewer ingredients listed on the label, the better. We also avoid fragrances in our skin-care products, as those can be irritating.

List of pore-clogging (comedogenic) ingredients:

Acetylated lanolin	Cetyl acetate
Acetylated lanolin alcohol	Chlorella
Algae extract	Chondrus crispus (aka Irish
Algin	moss or carageenan moss)
Butyl stearate	Coal tar
Carrageenan	Cocoa butter
Cetearyl alcohol +	Coconut alkanes
ceteareth-20	Coconut butter

Coconut oil
Colloidal sulfur
Cotton awws oil
Cottonseed oil
D&C Red #3
D&C Red #17
D&C Red #21
D&C Red #30
D&C Red #36
Decyl oleate
Dioctyl succinate
Disodium monooleamido
    PEG 2- sulfosuccinate
Ethoxylated lanolin
Ethylhexyl palmitate
Glyceryl stearate SE
Glyceryl-3 diisostearate
Hexadecyl alcohol
Hydrogenated vegetable oil
Isocetyl alcohol
Isocetyl stearate
Isodecyl oleate
Isopropyl isostearate
Isopropyl linolate
Isopropyl myristate
Isopropyl palmitate
Isostearyl isostearate
Isostearyl neopentanoate
Kelp
Laminaria digitata extract
Laminaria saccharina extract
    (laminaria saccharine)
Laureth-4
Laureth-23
Lauric acid
Mink oil
Myristic acid

Myristyl lactate
Myristyl myristate
Octyl palmitate
Octyl stearate
Oleth-3
Oleyl alcohol
PEG 8 stearate
PEG 16 lanolin
PEG 200 dilaurate
PG monostearate
Plankton
Polyglyceryl-3 diisostearate
Potassium chloride
PPG 2 myristyl propionate
Propylene glycol
    monostearate
Red algae
Seaweed
Sea whip extract
Shark liver oil
Shea
Shea butter
Sodium chloride
Sodium laureth sulfate
Sodium lauryl sulfate
Solulan 16
Sorbitan oleate
Soybean oil
Spirulina
Steareth 10
Stearic acid tea
Stearyl heptanoate
Sulfated castor oil
Sulfated jojoba oil
Wheat germ glyceride
Wheat germ oil
Xylene

You can also go to the Clear Skin Diet website at www.ClearSkinDiet.com and use the ingredients checker; enter ingredients and click "Check Ingredients" to see if any are pore clogging.

2. CLEANSE YOUR FACE LIKE YOU'RE AT A DAY SPA

"I already know how to wash my face." Actually, you may be overdrying your skin by washing it too often. The concept seems counterintuitive, but overdrying can make your face compensate by producing even more oil—just like over-shampooing your hair makes it more greasy.

You can't scrub the acne off your face, no matter how hard you try. In fact, the tougher you are on your skin, the more likely you are to aggravate it and make it break out even more. Your new job is to make your skin feel as pampered and spoiled as it would after a trip to a day spa—and you'll be doing this twice a day. Consider this as a "thank you" to your heroic skin for holding you together.

Before you wash your face with your cleanser, you're going to preclean your face with makeup-cleansing wipes (sans oil, of course). We recommend this for both men and women and regardless of whether or not you're wearing makeup. Gently remove any gook or grime from your skin with the wipe. Makeup-removal wipes are extremely soft, so you will not be in any danger of further irritating your skin. This may be enough for you. If you feel like you require additional cleansing, then wash your hands and pour a cleanser for acne-prone skin onto them and lather lightly. Apply the lather to your skin with your fingers, making very gentle circles around your face and neck. Take your time; this should feel good. Rinse with lukewarm water to remove cleanser. Cold or hot water can shock the skin and irritate it. Blot your face dry with a soft paper towel. Don't rub; blot. Guideline 5 explains why you probably want to choose paper towels over cloth. (See Appendix A: Recommended Products for suggested wipes and cleansers.)

3. MOISTURIZE ONLY IF YOU NEED IT

After you cleanse your skin at night, apply moisturizer only in the areas where you have dryness. You probably don't need to slather it all over your face. If your face is overly dry, then that may be an indicator that you are overwashing or overusing a topical. The solution to overdrying is not to add more topicals to your skin routine but to stop overusing the topicals that created the dry problem in the first place. Moisturize if you need it, just try your best not to overdo it. (See Appendix A: Recommended Products for compliant product suggestions.)

4. USE A MASK ONLY ONCE A WEEK

Once you are a couple of months into the program, you can (if you wish) add a mask to your routine one day a week (no more than that). Our recommended mask contains trace amounts of essential oil, though it is listed as non-comedogenic. The reason to wait a couple of months before trying it is that the mask might be an acne trigger for some people. Get your acne under control before introducing this mask or any other. Masks that contain charcoal or mud can tighten pores and dry up acne lesions. Don't use one of those ridiculous masks that are difficult to peel off your skin. You're not just removing oil with these masks, you're also taking off layers of your epidermis. These masks can also break capillaries in your skin. Stay away from these things; they are a dangerous gimmick. The mask we're recommending for limited use is Fresh Umbrian Clay Purifying Mask ("Fresh" is the company name), which contains trace amounts of sandalwood oil. Remember, you are waiting to use this mask a couple of months into your healing process and only if your acne is first clearing.

5. DRY YOUR FACE WITH PAPER TOWELS

We don't mean to gross you out by telling you this, but you may be sticking your face in something that's dirtier than your toilet bowl.

Your towels.

According to a May 2014 study done by the University of Arizona, the most bacteria-laden items in your home are towels. Eighty-nine percent of kitchen towels tested were infested with coliform bacteria, and 25 percent tested positive for *E. coli.*

When your face and body come in contact with towels, sheets, and pillowcases, you are leaving oil, dead skin cells, and other residues behind. You don't want to transfer that oil back onto your body when you come in contact with those items again. You should also not use a body towel on your face. Your arms, legs, shoulders, and armpits all have bacteria that are specific for those areas of the body. If you dry your armpits with a towel and then use it on your face—some of that special armpit bacteria will be moving onto your cheeks. Maybe you want to leave your armpit bacteria where it belongs, in your armpits.

We prefer blot drying our faces with paper towels; that way we don't have to remember to launder a washrag after each use. Some people might object to using paper products for environmental reasons, and we understand that. But laundering washcloths daily uses a fair amount of water, which isn't necessarily beneficial to the environment either. Soft paper towels are an easier solution. They are more hygienic than cloth, and you don't have to be concerned with installing some nasty bacteria onto your face each time you cleanse.

You also may want to consider changing your pillowcase every night, or sleeping on a clean towel over your pillow. You want your face to have a fresh, clean environment as you catch your winks.

Make sure your laundry detergent is non-comedogenic. We use unscented non-comedogenic laundry detergent from Costco ourselves. Your sheets, pillowcases, towels, washcloths, and clothing could all have a fine layer of film from your detergent, if it hasn't been completely rinsed off in your washing machine.

We haven't found any non-comedogenic fabric softeners and so are recommending against using softeners all together. (See Appendix A: Recommended Products to see some detergent recommendations.)

6. KEEP YOUR MAKEUP AND APPLICATORS CLEAN

Do you think dirty towels are gross? Wait until you hear about your makeup. If you don't clean your brushes and makeup regularly, they can get chock-full of bacteria, viruses, and fungi. Brimming! If you are struggling with acne, these beasties can cause even more acne or even a staph infection.

You can sterilize powdered makeup by spritzing it with a bit of alcohol and allowing it to dry. You can also use sterile sponges for dry or liquid makeup and dispose them after each use.

Makeup brushes can be washed with shampoo or an antibacterial soap and left to dry overnight. (See Appendix A: Recommended Products for brush cleaner recommendations.)

7. SPOT-TREAT BLEMISHES AND CYSTS

Before we even broach the topic of spot-treating any sort of acne, we'd like to remind you once again: *Don't pop pimples. Keep your hands off your face.* Once again: *Keep your hands off your face.* If you're not touching it, you're not tempted to pick at it.

Popping pimples pushes bacteria deeper into your skin and can even contribute to spreading bacteria to other parts of your face. It also takes longer for a popped pimple to heal and could lead to scarring.

To spot-treat a blemish, wash your face at night as previously instructed (we are going to ask you to limit spot treatment for nighttime to avoid additional irritation to your skin). Apply benzoyl peroxide or salicylic acid to spots only, not the entire face. Salicylic acid and benzoyl peroxide will help dry pimples.

For cysts, apply the following products in this order:

1. Salicylic acid (allow to dry)
2. Benzoyl peroxide (allow to dry)
3. Hydrocortisone cream (reduces inflammation)

If you really love having cysts on your face for months on end, then go ahead and try to pop them. You will be rewarded with pain and inflammation for weeks if you decide to try and pop a cyst—and possibly some big scars, too. If you would like the cyst to recede in a couple of days, try this method instead. (See Appendix A: Recommended Products.)

8. GET RID OF ACNE MECHANICA

There is actually another type of acne you may or may not have experienced. It's called acne mechanica, and is caused by excess heat, combined with friction and rubbing against the skin. Students (carrying heavy backpacks), athletes (wearing sports bras or athletic equipment), and soldiers (hauling heavy gear) are among those who experience acne mechanica. Purse straps and ill-fitting bras straps are also culprits. Here are some strategies for dealing with acne mechanica:

1. Loosen your bra straps.
2. Don't wear a backpack long enough to cause irritation—try shifting it around from time to time or even setting it down for periods to give your back a rest. Try not to put the backpack onto the same area once you start wearing it again.
3. Take your sweaty clothes off as quickly as you can after a workout, and don't put them back on again until they're laundered.
4. Try wearing natural fibers like cotton when you exercise, to allow your skin more of a chance to breathe.

If you have an acne mechanica breakout, first determine the source of the irritation (clothes, purse, whatever), and then treat the acne. Hydrocortisone cream is good for these types of breakouts, combined with an acne body wash.

9. PROTECT YOUR SKIN WITH SUNSCREEN

"But sunscreen makes me breakout!" Which do you hate more: a bad sunburn or a breakout? How about avoiding both? If you are planning on spending any time in the sun, wear sunscreen. Sunburns inflame acne and darken post-inflammatory hyperpigmentation (which we discuss in chapter 8). Many acne medications make the skin extra sun sensitive—an additional reason to make sure your skin is well shielded.

Sunburns can temporarily dry out the skin and cause it to peel. Remember what happens when your skin becomes overly dry? It produces more oil. More oil means potentially more acne.

10. CONCEAL WHILE YOU HEAL

Makeup. Love it, hate it, you wear it anyway. You think you can't live without it, so you hate it some more. We asked several of the participants in our Acne Intervention Programs their opinion about wearing makeup to camouflage breakouts, and their answers revealed some ambivalence. Some felt ashamed, embarrassed, and "fake" when they wore makeup to cover up their acne. But they still felt obligated to do so. Others didn't wear any makeup at all and felt guilty about that, too.

Here is our position on makeup: if you feel more confident when you hide your pimples, then go ahead and do *not* feel any guilt or psychic discomfort about doing so. If you don't feel comfortable wearing makeup, then don't do it—and don't let anyone pressure you otherwise. The truth is, there are good arguments for concealing and there are also good reasons to let your skin just breathe. Be comfortable whether your wear it or not. As it's such a personal matter, this decision needs to be left up to you.

This section is for those who fall into the "hide every damn spot" camp. You want to conceal while you heal? Well, we totally support that! For us, our ability to more or less effectively cover severe breakouts helped us maintain our sanity. We get it. You know the acne is there, but maybe you don't want it to be so obvious to others. That's totally cool, really. While your skin is going through its healing process, you officially have permission to make every zit disappear as much as you can.

Nina and I practically grew up performing onstage and learned to apply makeup when we were pretty young. There is a bit of an art form to hiding pimples well, though. So we're going to share some acne-concealing tips we've learned so that you can help your breakouts do a big vanishing act.

We do have some recommendations about products to use for each of these steps, but we'd like you to bear in mind how difficult it is to find makeup products that are perfect. There may be one or two ingredients in your makeup that are not ideal. We are about 99 percent behind the products we are recommending; with makeup, you may have to compromise some (do not compromise on highly comedogenic ingredients, obviously). Unfortunately, it's a lot easier to control what you put into your mouth than what you put on your face.

First, cleanse your face as we've previously detailed. You want to start with a fresh "palette." You don't want to apply makeup to less than clean skin. It's not good for your skin, and the makeup will not adhere properly.

Next, apply powder lightly with a brush to soak up excess oil. One powder we like is Nyx Studio Finishing Powder.

Next step is to apply a matte primer. A good primer is a fabulous tool to keep in your makeup arsenal. It does a few things: your makeup will apply more easily, excess oils will be soaked up, and it acts as a barrier between the foundation and your skin. Your makeup will stay smoother and in place longer if you apply a good primer first. One primer we like is called Smash Box Photo Finish More Than Primer.

Now the next thing you want to do is apply a green concealer stick. Uh... wait—did you say *green*? I know it sounds weird, but if you are covering up acne, you want to use a green concealer stick over the spots. Green helps neutralize the red and cover up the irritation. If you don't have redness, you don't need to use a green concealer; you can use a regular concealer. Blot onto skin with a clean makeup sponge. We're going to recommend a product for this called Au Naturale Color Theory Crème Corrector in Sweet Basil.

Now it's time to apply your foundation. Once you have covered up active red spots with the green concealer, apply foundation with clean spongers over the concealer. Use a combination dabbing-wiping motion, and make sure your entire face is covered. Blend into the neck, so you don't have an infamous makeup line at your jaw line. We're going to recommend a foundation called Tarte Amazonian Clay 12-Hour Full Coverage Foundation SPF-15.

The final step is to dust with finishing powder to set the makeup. Go forth with confidence!

◇

Skin-Care Cheat Sheet

Use gentle, oil-free products.

Read skin- and hair-care ingredients carefully.

Cleanse skin like you're at a day spa.

Moisturize only as necessary.

Change towels and pillowcases often.

Use non-comedogenic laundry detergent.

Use sunscreen.

—◇—

DIET STOPS ACNE: RACHEL LEONARD, AGE 28

Dealing with acne in high school is almost expected, but graduating college and planning a wedding with a face full of painful, cystic acne was one of the most depressing and defeating experiences Rachel Leonard said she ever experienced. Despite eating a plant-based diet and running the gamut of conventional treatments (birth control, anti-inflammatory medicine, antibiotics, topicals, and even Accutane), Rachel found that her acne would always return, each time coming back stronger and more persistent.

Rachel was watching a presentation by Dr. John McDougall when he told our story—how we had eaten a clean plant-based diet and had gotten rid of our severe acne by eliminating specific foods and skin products. Rachel immediately identified with our experiences; she signed up for our acne Intervention pilot study and followed it to a T. She was amazed with the almost immediate changes, not only in how her skin looked but also in how it felt. A few months in was the first time in a long time that Rachel could wash her face and not feel a bump, scab, or rough patch. Rachel says she is enjoying the new sense of self that has been restored after a decade of fighting what most of her friends had kicked after puberty. Rachel wrote: "There are no words to express my gratitude for Nina and Randa's decision to share their story. I can only hope to make an impact on someone else's life by now sharing mine."

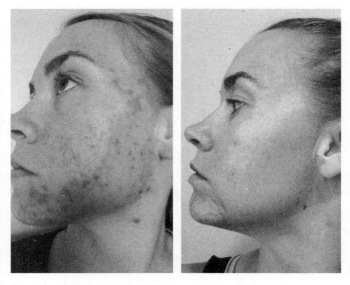

(See color photos in insert.)

8

ACNE SPOTS, SCARS, AND INTERVENTIONS

by Randa

"When you have acne, you keep thinking about how ugly it is and how everyone is just looking at it all the time—and it makes it so much worse!"

—Bella Thorne

Sometimes you feel like the acne saga will never end. You finally have cleared up your acne, but it looks like you still have acne. What's up with that? Not to worry, we've got your back on this, too. Just read on.

A participant in one of our Acne Intervention Programs had succeeded in arresting her acne. She had no new breakouts, no whiteheads or blackheads, and her face had finally calmed down and begun the healing process. She was disappointed, though. Her acne had lessened, but she still had these small red marks on her face in the area where her acne had been active. The spots weren't on top of her skin, and they weren't scars—there were no real bumps or indentations. The discoloration seemed like it was just under the skin. She wondered if her acne was somehow still active, even though she hadn't had any breakouts in weeks. Was this even acne? And could she do anything about it?

The answers are: it is not acne, and she can work on the spots. These small red spots have a technical name: post-inflammatory hyperpigmentation (PIH). PIH are areas where your skin becomes darkened or pink or brown tinted. They manifest as spots or patches of color on your face, or in places where you've had acne. This is not acne scarring. PIH is a relatively smooth area where there is a darker color underneath but no active acne causing it. PIH is a result of inflammation from acne that changed the skin tone just under the dermis, and the tone has not returned to its normal color.

The good news is PIH will recede over time, even without any treatment. For some people, it might only take a few weeks or months for the color to decrease and present as normal skin again. But in others, the pigmentation can take up to twenty-four months to fully disappear. The length of time depends on how much darker the spot is compared to the rest of your skin tone. The darker the spot, the longer it's going to take. The key to overcoming PIH is simply patience. There are no quick fixes for this problem, so you might as well relax and forget about those darn spots. They will eventually disappear.

Whether or not you opt to actively treat your PIH spots, you can do several things to minimize the redness. One is to avoid washing your face with anything that irritates your skin. If you inflame your skin, you're inhibiting your progress. One of the first lines of defense for PIH is to cleanse with a 2.5 percent benzoyl peroxide. (See Appendix A: Recommended Products for some suggestions.)

You can also help minimize the appearance of your PIH spots by using sunscreen. Sunburns increase the contrast of color between PIH spots and your natural skin tone, making them more visible. Light from the UV spectrum can make PIH take longer to fade. Sunscreen is also critical because many of the following treatments make your skin more sun sensitive. Many dermatologists recommend you use a sunscreen of at least 30 SPF. Make sure you get a sunscreen that is non-comedogenic—meaning it will not block your pores. This is crucial. If sunscreen clogs your pores, you could be saying hello to the acne you just said good-bye to. Choose a sunscreen that's made for breakout-prone skin.

TREATMENTS FOR PIH SPOTS

Can anything be done to expedite fading? Yes. But first, you want to make sure your acne is under control and you don't have active acne. Once the acne has ceased, then you can start to explore ways to deal with PIH spots.

Now to be honest, strategies that work for one person may not work for another. The most reliable solution is time. You will need to experiment with your PIH, and have patience to learn your best course of action. When our acne cleared, Nina and I both had PIH marks. We initially tried various strategies, but eventually decided to cover them with makeup, since that's easy. Our PIH spots disappeared completely within six months. We haven't personally tried most of the following strategies, but we did research about what worked for others with PIH. You need to understand that even with these treatments and approaches, it may take significant time for your PIH spots to fade.

OVER-THE-COUNTER BRIGHTENING PRODUCTS

There are brightening treatment products that can help with mild PIH spots. People we know who have tried them tell us that they are a waste of money. They apparently don't work for everyone; they may or may not work for you. Most of these treatments contain a combination of alpha and beta hydroxyl acids (BHA), u glycolic acid, vitamin A, vitamin C, or other ingredients intended to exfoliate the skin. Avoid products that break down the skin in any way, such as scrubs with small hard particles or a hard-surfaced product that scrapes your face. We recommend using Paula's Choice RESIST Brightening Essence.

Hydroquinone is another brightening product, often used to treat PIH. Hydroquinone is an organic compound that can cause a condition called ochronosis, where skin becomes tough and actually darkens. Hydroquinone is banned in Japan, the EU, and Australia. Frankly, we wouldn't use it ourselves. We are going to leave this decision up to you and recommend proceeding with much caution. As an over-the-counter product, it's available at 1 to 2 percent strength, but you can get higher strengths by prescription. It often contains other ingredients that are supposed to give improved results. The creams are applied only on the darker areas, and you have to be careful not to put them on your regular skin because you could end up lightening it, as well. Also, some people get skin irritation from these products. Obviously, if anything irritates your face, stop.

AZELAIC ACID

This product is available only by prescription and works by decreasing inflammation and speeding up cell turnover rates. If you don't want to use hydroquinone, this is another option to consider. Like many prescription topicals, there can be unwelcome side effects, such as itching, burning, stinging, tingling, tenderness, and dryness, so again, proceed with some caution. Dermatologists do find azelaic acid to be helpful in many cases and may prescribe it as part of a treatment regime. If you use it, just keep a careful eye out for redness or irritation.

VITAMIN C SERUM

This serum is another common treatment for dark spots and sun damage. Used in higher concentration, it's thought to brighten the skin and is sometimes used to lighten scar tissue. This has fewer negative side effects than other options. We recommend Amara Organics C Serum.

PHOTOFACIAL/IPS PROCEDURES

These procedures are done in a clinic, administered by a dermatologist. The dermatologist shoots intense pulsing light into the red or darker PIH areas, which breaks up discoloration. This procedure is more expensive, of course, but if you need fast results, it may be a good option. It may work in as little as two weeks, but it also may require three to five treatments to get results. Check recommendation services like Living Social and Groupon for discounted services.

CHEMICAL PEELS AND MICRODERMABRASION

Your dermatologist will probably have a number of other more aggressive options, such as peels, to deal with PIH. Again, this would normally require a series of treatments and need to be undertaken by a medical professional.

If you've successfully used the Clear Skin Diet to heal your acne but have some residual PIH spots, take comfort that you've halted the source of your problem. Over time these spots will recede.

TREATMENTS FOR ACNE SCARS

Once you've been able to halt new breakouts and "turn off" your acne, your skin starts to heal, inflammation calms, and now you can see what your face really looks like without active acne. If you've had a severe or prolonged bout with acne, you may have scarring, anything from mild unevenness to pockmarks and deep gouges.

There are two basic kinds of acne scars: scars caused by a loss of tissue and scars caused by an excess of new tissue. Acne is temporary, but scars can be permanent. When acne is modest and occurring near the skin's surface, the resulting lesion is usually manageable. When acne is deeper and more intense, destroying deeper or larger areas of healthy skin tissue, your skin forms new collagen fibers to repair the wound. Collagen is a strong and somewhat rigid protein that covers the injured area, and the collagen "repair job" often leaves the skin a lot less smooth than it was before. This is an acne scar. Sometimes your body produces too much collagen, and the result is a mass of raised tissue on your face. This type of scar is called hypertrophic or keloid scars. The other more common type of scarring is caused by depressed scars, where there has been a loss of tissue. "Ice pick" and "boxcar" are names for scars created by such a depression.

While you're breaking out, you want to reduce inflammation as much as possible to prevent the blemish from doing permanent damage to the skin. We know you've heard this before, but we're going to say it again: *keep your hands off your face.* Never squeeze, pop, or pick at pimples. This can cause the infection in a pimple to spread and make inflammation worse. Popping pimples will extend the healing time and increases the chance of leaving a permanent scar. And don't pick at scabs either. A scab is a "bandage" the skin creates to protect healing. Again, removing a scab will only extend the healing time.

There is a wide range of treatments available for acne scars. We aren't going to try to cover all of them but will touch on some of the best-known and most commonly used approaches. Obviously, if you have acne scars you want to remove, you should talk to your dermatologist or other skin professional to determine which options are best for you.

EXFOLIATION AND DERMABRASION BRUSHES

Over-the-counter exfoliators include buff puffs or pumice stones, or face washes with small particles. Dermabrasion brushes have spinning brushes with bristles, which remove dead skin to help prevent further clogging. These are modest approaches that may help with modest scarring but probably won't be very effective for more significant scarring.

RETIN-A

Retin-A is a prescription topical ointment derived from vitamin A. Retin-A can be successful for modest scars and overall skin texture, as well as fading dark spots. It causes skin cells to turn over more rapidly and shrinks dilated pores. It also boosts collagen production, which helps smooth skin and soften creases or wrinkles.

CHEMICAL PEELS

A dermatologist can apply chemical peels in their office. After cleaning your skin, they will apply chemicals—such as glycolic acid, trichloroacetic acid, salicylic acid, lactic acid, or carbolic acid—to your face or the area being treated. This injures the skin, making it blister. Over the next week or two, the dead skin peels away, exposing new, softer skin. There are different levels of peels, from gentle to very powerful; the latter requires more recovery time and can be uncomfortable while the chemicals are applied. You will appear to have a sunburn and will need to stay out of the sun and use sunblock regularly for several months to protect the new skin. Some people have found chemical peels to be very useful. They can usually be repeated in six to twelve months.

MICRODERMABRASION AND LASER TREATMENTS

Microdermabrasion and laser treatments are for deeper or more serious acne scarring. These can be very expensive, but they can also work wonders. Microdermabrasion employs a machine that shoots small crystals into your skin while another section of the machine vacuums up the particles. The crystals are shot into your skin at a uniform depth, damaging the skin evenly. This can be a little painful. Collagen production is stimulated as the skin tries to heal, smoothing out pocks and depressions somewhat.

Laser treatments work the same way. Several different kinds of lasers damage your skin and make the pits and pocks heal up around the same height as the rest of the skin. The process you choose depends on your particular skin and the issues you need to correct. Generally, multiple treatments are required over time to get a good result, and that can run into the thousands of dollars. The latest entry to this class of treatment is the picosecond laser, which stimulates collagen production by triggering changes in cellular behavior. One picosecond-laser treatment can cost between $600 and $1,500.

DERMAPEN

Dermapen is another procedure that deliberately injures your skin, using microneedles, which causes microinjuries to the epidermis and dermis. The microinjuries encourage and harness your body's innate ability to repair the skin. The Dermapen is similar to a tattoo gun. The pen is rubbed over your face, injuring both the acne scars and normal skin and stimulating collagen production to, once again, stimulate the skin to heal up at an even level. You will probably have to repeat the process a number of times to get the desired result, and it sometimes takes many months of healing before your skin starts to normalize. It's considerably less expensive than laser treatments.

FILLERS AND AUGMENTATIONS

Fillers and augmentations are perhaps the most invasive processes and most costly. Your dermatologist will stick needles into the skin, free the skin from the dermis below, and pump in fillers to remove the pocks and valleys from areas that are depressed on the face. The skin will be smoothed to the same level. The amount of treatment you may require depends on the amount of damage to be repaired. The more severe your scarring, the more dramatic and expensive the repair will be.

Consult with your own doctor but get opinions from different doctors. Some doctors recommend a particular method because they own that machine, and so that's what they would rather do. Request before and after photos and examples of the results you can reasonably expect.

Although the more significant treatments can get expensive, frequently there are specials on Groupon or Living Social or other coupon-style web services, where you can get access to many of these services at highly discounted rates. If you have used these services before, you know that you can check out reviews on the Groupon website or Yelp or other online review sites. Many major, reputable dermatologists will have these offers from time to time, in order to bring in new business. Try to find deals to make these options more affordable. Remind yourself that you have probably by this point already saved thousands of dollars in acne products by choosing the Clear Skin Diet over prescriptions, so you may be able to spend your money now where you really need it—to be rid of any acne memories your skin might still be holding onto.

GOOD THINGS COME TO THOSE WHO PERSEVERE

Brian Turner, whose acne story you read at the end of chapter 3, had severe acne for many years. His acne scarring was acute. When Brian changed his diet and disrupted new acne breakouts, his face finally began to heal. He says it took a year for his PIH spots to completely fade. Then he began researching ways to deal with scarring. He experimented with dermabrasion and other strategies. It took another nine months to finally see the great results of his dermabrasion.

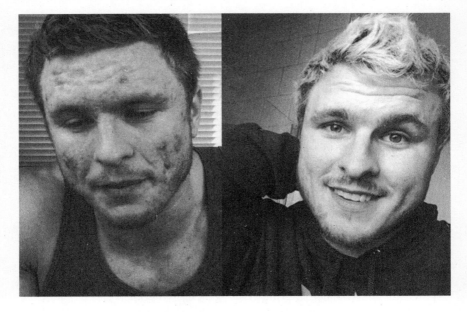

It took Brian two years of effort to go from the photo on the left, with lots of active acne, PIH, and scarring, to the right where he is today—looking like a new person, and leaving the legacy of acne behind him. (You can watch videos of Brian's actual microdermabrasion and other treatments on his YouTube channel; see Resources.)

Nina and I had fairly dramatic and quick improvement, probably because we hadn't been afflicted with severe acne for very long. Many people have acne for years at the level we had for a few months. We'd had some extreme flare-ups for about six months before we embarked on this diet. Experiencing severe acne for a relatively short period of time meant less opportunity for deep damage, injury, or scarring. Someone who has been battling serious acne for many years will probably require more intensive recovery approaches, as Brian Turner did.

The sooner you change your diet, the sooner you can get your acne under control. Then you can begin the process of dealing with scarring, or any other issues caused by the acne.

—◇—

DIET STOPS ACNE: KATARINA LEISER, AGE 24

Katarina had struggled with painful, cystic acne since she was ten years old. She was the only person in her elementary school with acne. In the sixth grade, she learned to hide her face with her hands and hair.

Katarina's cystic acne was so painful it hurt to lie on her pillow at night. Two dermatologists recommended she try Accutane, but she felt her acne must have to do with diet. She found our YouTube videos on acne and diet and felt even more certain her acne must be food related. She applied to be in one of our Acne Intervention Programs and cleared her acne in three months. Katarina is now coping with scarring and PIH, which requires more time to be repaired, but she said she is ecstatic that she has no more breakouts. When Katarina traveled to Los Angeles, she contacted us, and we had the pleasure of meeting her in person.

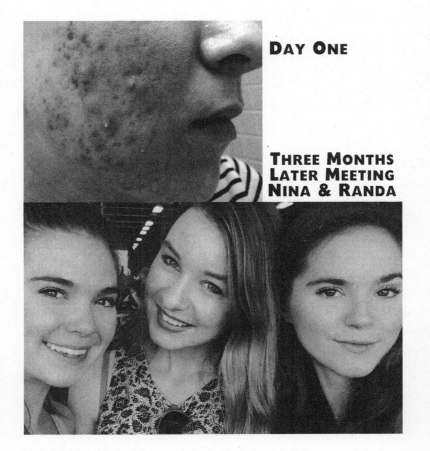

DAY ONE

THREE MONTHS LATER MEETING NINA & RANDA

9

ACNE HURTS: EMOTIONAL SCARRING

by Nina

"The prevalence [of acne vulgaris] is highest in adolescence, where the individual counters several psychosocial changes...In different studies, presence of some mental disorders in patients with acne was reported, including low self-esteem, avoidance, hastiness and anxiety, depression, shame, suicidal thoughts and attempts, and difficulties in applying for a job."

—Javad Golchai, MD[1]

A study of the prevalence of anxiety and depression showed that 25 percent of acne patients suffered with depression and about 70 percent with anxiety.[2] I think that anxiety number is probably closer to 100 percent. I haven't met anyone yet who feels joyful about a breakout. I know I never did. That day I told my mom that I felt like Robin Williams was a real low point for me, a low point several months in the making. And this feeling of desperate sadness that my twenty-year-old self was experiencing was because of my severe acne.

When my acne was at its worst, I basically shut my life down. I stopped seeing friends, going to the gym, dancing, and working on my career. I was merely waiting for it to go away so I could start my life again. We heard very similar stories from nearly everyone who enrolled in our Acne Intervention Programs. The emotionally painful isolation imposed by the physically painful acne is perhaps the most difficult thing our program participants deal with. I completely relate.

In February 2015, the British Skin Foundation commissioned a survey about how acne impacts a person's mental health. The survey was the largest they had ever done, and they received over two thousand responses. The results of this survey are sobering:

- ✧ 20 percent of acne sufferers surveyed had contemplated suicide. That's one in five.
- ✧ 57 percent had been verbally abused by friends, family members, or others.
- ✧ 10 percent felt they had been unfairly fired.
- ✧ 20 percent had a relationship end due to their acne.

Acne can obviously have a profound effect. Dermatologist and British Skin Foundation spokesperson Dr. Anjali Mahto, commenting on this survey said, "I think these results highlight that acne should be taken far more seriously."

Prior to our acne crisis, I would have described myself as happy, confident, and well-adjusted. The months of severe acne chipped away at my confidence until I felt like a shell of my former self. Although getting rid of my acne contributed greatly to my mental health recovery, Randa and I also started coming out of our depression before the acne disappeared. The following are thoughts about some of what people with acne deal with.

ISOLATION

Self-imposed isolation is probably the number-one complaint we heard about from people with friends who suffer with acne. This problem seems to be universal. It's perfectly healthy to spend some time in solitude. In fact, it's probably beneficial. But social isolation is something else entirely. Whatever problem you are experiencing can be amplified when you don't have anyone to talk to, when depressive thoughts are given free rein to bounce around in your head. Social isolation can be a result of shame, depression, or low self-worth—all of which can be caused by acne because you don't want to be seen. How do we overcome this desire to hide away until the acne clears up?

BULLYING

A survey sponsored by Galderma Laboratories, L.P., of 817 teenagers indicated that teenagers with acne were more likely to be bullied than those without (76 percent versus 53 percent). Just what you need, right? You're already feeling self-conscious and nervous about your appearance, and then someone decides to be hurtful and insult you. Bodybuilder Brian Turner talked about being bullied in high school for his acne; when someone makes fun of something that people don't have any control over, that says everything about the bully and nothing about you.

Brian said bullying about acne can get downright vicious. On his YouTube channel about fitness, Brian used to encounter comments like "Eww, your face! I was eating! I got nauseous looking at you!" People normally don't say something like this to someone who has a receding hairline or is overweight. This is the kind of bullying reserved for people with acne. Brian says to never let these kinds of people bring you down. Never ever allow yourself to think, "I'm not a worthwhile person." And try your best not to react to bullies; they are simply trying to get a reaction, to engage. Ignoring is always the best, or reporting their bullying to someone in authority. Reporting a bully also may protect someone else from the bully. Remember that bullies are not happy people. Well-adjusted people who are content with their own lives don't want to cause pain for others.

SELF-ESTEEM

My sister and I had supportive family and friends during our acne crisis, and our self-esteem still took a major hit. One thing my mom did that actually made me feel better was to research various celebrities who had also had severe acne. She texted me photos of Cameron Diaz, Megan Fox, Katy Perry, Keira Knightley, and Lorde. These are all incredibly talented and powerful women, whom I

ACNE ADVICE:
From Rip Esselstyn

How badly do you want it? If you truly want to eliminate your acne and live your healthiest life, draw a line in the sand and don't cross over it. Focus on those fruits, vegetables, whole intact grains, and the amazing legumes that are out there and skip the overtly fat plant foods. Commit 100 percent to eating a low-fat, whole food, plant-strong diet. It's not a huge sacrifice—don't let your mind trick you into thinking it is! You are completely and totally worth making this change. Once your acne starts to disappear and your skin starts to clear up, you'll be jumping to the moon and back with joy and staying compliant will be an afterthought. It will just become part of who you are now—bring it on!

admire. She said very bluntly, "They are not quitting their jobs and letting acne prevent them from pushing forward with their lives. You're not going to let that happen either." Knowing that these women decided to set aside their insecurities and persevere anyway and were ultimately successful made me want to do the same.

If your self-esteem has taken a nosedive because of acne, do your best to persevere. Keep moving forward. This is the number-one way to rebuild and keep your self-esteem. Be who you are *right now*, not who you'll imagine you'll be on the day your skin clears up.

Here are a few things to consider as you move forward to help stay positive and maximize your motivation.

FIND A CLEAR SKIN DIET FRIEND

One of the most helpful things you can do is to find a friend or family member who will do the program with you. Nothing is better than having a support system. When we first started talking on YouTube about how we healed our acne through diet, lots of people posted comments about trying it themselves. They asked us for advice, and suggested the kinds of videos they wanted us to make. Then an interesting thing started happening. People in the comments section started talking with one another about the diet, comparing notes, asking questions, sharing their own recipes and cooking strategies. A support community started taking shape in the comments section under our acne videos. We realized that interacting with other people who are doing this diet is inspiring.

In running our first small pilot study of the Clear Skin Diet, we found that doing the program with other people is almost a spiritual experience. Everyone made a deep connection, while sharing ideas and strategies. At the end of each Tuesday night meeting, we practically had to kick everyone out of the meeting room because we were having such a good time. No one wanted to leave. Even then, most of us would stand around outside in the parking lot and continue chatting. We also hosted a private Facebook group, where there was also a lot of mutual support.

When starting the Clear Skin Diet, see if you can find an acne support group, or create one on your own. That can have big benefits. Convincing a friend or family member (or two!) to do it with you is going to make it much easier and help set you up for long-term success. If you don't have a friend with acne, there are other reasons they might want to join you, like weight loss. Don't limit yourself to asking friends with acne to join you.

FIND OTHER RESOURCES

If you can't find a friend to do it with, then find a book, website, or group that can offer support. Obviously, we recommend our own book and website as resources, but there are additional books you might enjoy. We recommend reading *The Starch Solution, The Healthiest Diet on the Planet,* or *The McDougall Program for Maximum Weight Loss*—all by John McDougall, MD. (Of course, you may have to customize some recipes slightly if they contain avocados or any of the higher-fat plant foods, but basically the McDougalls have amazingly wonderful, healthy recipes.) Any of the books by Rip Esselstyn (*The Engine 2 Diet*) or his father Caldwell Esselstyn Jr., MD (*Prevent and Reverse Heart Disease*), and all of the *Forks Over Knives* books. Immersing yourself in the knowledge, science, and approaches of top plant-based experts is a great way to reinforce your decision and to stay strong and motivated going forward.

DEALING WITH SETBACKS

By the way, you might misstep. You might find yourself in a situation you weren't prepared for and you eat something you know you didn't want to eat. Or you find yourself somewhere and just craving something you know won't help your face, but for whatever reason you couldn't resist. We have one message if that happens: don't beat yourself up. The Clear Skin Diet is about getting your acne under control and moving forward in the healthiest version of you possible. But if you slip up at some point, just forgive yourself, pick up where you left off, and move ahead.

One of our Acne Intervention Program participants, Fatima Carrera, shared with the group that she had attended a friend's birthday party after work because the friend told her she had some baked potatoes for Fatima. Before Fatima arrived, someone else had already eaten all the potatoes. There was nothing "legal" for Fatima to eat. Starved, Fatima decided to eat "just a few" potato chips... and ended up eating more than a few. She said she felt terrible and could feel the grease on her face building up. She broke out within about a day and was really upset. Fatima learned that day that she needed to plan ahead better and anticipate situations like this. Bring your own food, or else just stop somewhere and eat before going somewhere where there may be nothing for you to eat. You don't want to find yourself starving with no good options so always plan ahead. And if you do deviate from the Clear Skin Diet, don't sweat it. Just do a mental reboot; remember tomorrow's a new day and start again.

CLEAR SKIN MIND-SET

One of the brilliant and inspiring experts we consulted in writing this book is psychiatrist and bestselling author Walter Jacobson, MD. Dr. Jacobson was involved in our acne interventions and worked to inspire participants. He was very direct in advice he had for people battling acne and the accompanying emotional challenges. Here is what Dr. Jacobson shared about the psychology of success on the Clear Skin Diet:

ACNE ADVICE:
From Walter Jacobson, MD

Affirm what you want. Visualize it with intensity and passion. If it's your acne being healed, picture that. Turn off the negative thinking. Turn off the inner critic. Turn off the name-calling of yourself—"I'm ugly. I'm useless. No one likes me." Tune out people who are telling you, "Oh, what's the big deal? You should just get over it." Have the courage to not care what other people think or say about you. You deserve happiness and success, so don't allow anyone to derail you. It will serve you well to use this program to learn how to be fearless. Learn how to not let the judgments, the attitudes, even the body language of other people interfere with who you are and how you feel about yourself.

Motivation is key. We remind ourselves daily why we are doing this diet. We remind ourselves that there is delayed gratification with anything worth accomplishing. We remind ourselves that there will be a great payoff at the end of this process. Our skin will be markedly improved. Additionally, we will be happier, healthier, more confident and more self-assured.

Also remember that success is a process of two steps forward and one step back. So when we fall back into old behaviors, we don't beat ourselves up. We don't call ourselves names. We don't perceive ourselves to be losers or failures. We recognize that setbacks aren't actually setbacks. They are stepping-stones to success. And we get back to our game plan with the motivation and commitment to keep at it until we achieve our goal.

Another tip for staying compliant is shutting off our inner critic. The inner critic is a voice inside our head which is very negative, pessimistic, and cynical. It puts us down. It calls us names. It tells us people don't really like us. It tells us what we're trying to do isn't worth doing. Or it isn't possible. Or no matter how hard we try we will fail. That it's pointless to try because nothing will ever change.

We need to shut down that inner critic, that negative voice. We give it no power. We tell it to shut up and go away, go haunt somebody else, we don't need or want its negativity. And we replace that inner critic with our inner colleague, a part of ourselves that is wise and true, and knows what's best for us. When we are calm and quiet, we can access that inner colleague for the nurturing, support, and wisdom that we need.

We also need to shut off negativity from others. There may be people who are family and friends, who want the best for us, but who also may be threatened by our desire for change and growth. And they may say things, subtle comments that are unconsciously designed to derail us from our program. We need to be aware of that and have our radar up for those sorts of comments so they don't discourage us and influence us to give up.

We tell ourselves that acne is not eternity. That this is not forever. That this diet works, and if we diligently work it, it will work for us. We remind ourselves that it will take time, and so we need to have faith, be patient, and persist.

We encourage ourselves not to let the depression of having bad acne cause us to hide in our room, to isolate ourselves and avoid friends and family. This only makes us more depressed. It is bad enough that we have been victimized, so to speak, by a physical condition. By banishing ourselves from the rest of the world, we victimize ourselves even further.

When we are ashamed and embarrassed by the way we look, we remind ourselves that this is a physical condition that says nothing about who we are as human beings, as loving souls on the planet deserving of love, happiness, and success.

—◇—

One more thing you should know: your decision to pick up this book and be willing to try something radically different to improve your life says something very positive about you. You want to take control of your skin, your body, your life. Think about how incredibly empowering that is. You're taking the time to educate yourself and make happier food choices. You can transfer this kind of mentality to just about any aspect of your life you want to improve.

—◇—

DIET STOPS ACNE: CATCHING UP

So many people on YouTube told us they followed our diet and got rid of their acne. We wanted to follow up and find out how they were doing six months after getting rid of their acne with the diet. Here were some responses:

> Before I made the switch I was actually vegetarian. And I
> ate a LOT of cheese! Like mac and cheese every day and

cereal with whole milk. Since discovering your channel and changing, I've been eating much more starchy foods like sweet potatoes and rice. I eat very low fat but occasionally I'll eat vegan ice cream or guacamole. As far as my skin goes, it's worked wonders for me! And I used to always feel congested and more tired, but now I have a lot more energy and no runny nose. I recommend to everybody everything you guys put out about diet. It has helped me so much; I would never switch back.

—Miriam, age nineteen

Before changing my diet I used to eat a lot of cottage cheese, Greek yogurt, meat, nuts, some veggies, and chickpeas. I guess you could say I was "paleo" because essentially I was afraid of carbs! I started taking your advice in October of 2015 and have been eating lots of various types of rice, potatoes, veggies, and fruit. The diet totally worked for me. My acne had been out of control and has now subsided completely. I've also lost eight pounds. And I used to have extremely irregular and painful periods, but now it's the complete opposite. I am totally eating this way for life!

—Angela, age twenty-one

I was actually vegan for about six months before trying the very low fat diet you guys recommend. I was still eating processed veggie "meats" fried in coconut oil, french fries, oily soups, vegan cheese pizzas, vegan chocolate, peanut and other nut butters, and salad dressings with oil. I now eat a lot of rice, beans, lentils, pasta, fruit, salads, and potato fries, which I make myself in the oven with no oil. I want to thank you guys. I would have never tried out this diet, and it has really improved my skin. It hasn't just helped my skin; it has also helped with my digestion and the way I feel. I feel full but never weighed down. This diet is actually treating the cause of my acne. And it has absolutely NO side effects besides looking and feeling your best!

—Carly, age twenty

PART III

TAKING ACTION

10

CLEAR SKIN LIVING STRATEGIES

by Randa

The Clear Skin Diet is a six-week program to empower you to change your diet and heal your skin. It might take some people more than six weeks, and that's OK. You need to give your body enough time to understand and get accustomed to the program. We don't want people to try the Clear Skin Diet, see solid improvements emerging, and then slip back into some of their old ways and trigger problems again.

This part of the book is to give you tools to help you make the Clear Skin Diet part of your routine. We want it to become such a normal part of your lifestyle that you don't have to think about it at all. This is just the way you live. The strategies ahead are meant to set you up for sustainability.

ACNE ADVICE:
From Ann Esselstyn

Eating plant based may feel challenging at first, but if you stick to the guidelines, your taste will change. Pizza without cheese becomes delicious. Oily salad dressings of the past are unthinkable. Banana soft serve from a Yonana machine topped with raspberry sauce and a sprinkle of chocolate balsamic vinegar is sweetly delicious. And if you are at all like us, rice and beans with all the fixings become your favorite meal and not only a favorite any night (every night?) meal but maybe like us even your special company meal. But there are endless fabulous possibilities. It is such fun to take a recipe you love and adapt it to whole food plant-based nutrition.

EAT!

Some of the most common challenges people may experience when switching to the Clear Skin Diet can arise from simply not eating enough. The food you're going to be consuming is less processed, lower in calories, and contains ample fiber and bulk. If you don't eat enough calories, you may not feel satisfied. If this happens to you, eat larger portions or more often. When you feel hungry, eat. Don't worry about whether you ate two hours ago, or what time you may want to eat. Hungry at midnight? Eat at midnight. As you get used to the Clear Skin Diet, try to trust your body's natural hunger signals. You won't overeat on a natural, whole food, plant-based diet. Crave more baked fries? Then have more! Definitely make sure you are eating enough starches. Foods like potatoes and rice provide satiety and fullness that can last. Eating enough good food will help crowd out the desire for the foods you used to eat, which gave you acne.

THE MICROWAVE IS NOT YOUR ENEMY

Some people are absolutely convinced that microwaves are satanic nuclear devices. They believe microwaves destroy the nutrition in food and introduce radiation into it and that they'll grow an extra set of fingers if they eat microwaved food. Is any of that true? Well, one of the most esteemed plant-based nutritionists, Jeff Novick, MS, RD, has researched and written extensively on the subject over many years. Jeff concluded that microwaves are about as dangerous as your electric toothbrush. Meaning you won't grow an extra set of anything if you use one.

Michael Greger, MD, is a popular vegan physician and best-selling author who specializes in reviewing and reporting on published medical literature. Whenever he examines a subject, he reads every study available from all angles to see where the truth most likely lays. After extensive reviews of numerous microwave studies, Dr. Greger concluded that a microwave is one of the most efficient cooking methods available and that it has virtually no impact on a food's nutrients. Dr. Greger reported that the shorter cooking times of microwave ovens actually preserve more nutrients than any other cooking method. And there's nothing radioactive about warming or cooking your food in a microwave.

All this means is that taking leftovers from your fridge and warming them up in the microwave is one of the easiest and best ways to prepare a truly healthy meal. So "nuke" away!

GO AHEAD AND BE LAZY—LIKE US!

You don't have to spend a bunch of time making elaborate recipes or fancy meals. We sometimes buy prepared rice, which can be frozen or unfrozen rice that has already been cooked and is packaged and sold in small portions. My mom calls it "bachelor rice" because it's so easy that any cooking-impaired single guy can make it. But that's probably sexist! If we're in a hurry or just feeling tired, we'll sometimes buy precooked rice and zap it in the microwave for some fast rice. Or we stick in a spud and press "potato" or microwave at full power for five minutes, microwave some frozen veggies next, open a can of beans and warm 'em up, add some ketchup or salsa or just plain old salt— and yum! This is a basic, quick, easy, and very satisfying clear skin meal. And to be honest, we very often eat this way. You can improve this meal or any other by getting creative with herbs and spices—they can dramatically liven up just about any meal. Experiment and be sure to keep your favorite spices on hand.

KEEP HEALTHY SNACKS AVAILABLE

We agree with Jeff Novick: snacks are just smaller amounts of any compliant food that you already eat and enjoy.

ACNE ADVICE:
From Rip Esselstyn

You can't beat fresh fruit and veggies for snacking, but there are some really great options out there for when you want something different or you're in a pinch.

- Everybody loves chips and salsa, but there's really not many compliant chips out there. So buy some corn tortillas (fat-free) and bake them in the oven: they make incredibly tasty chips. There's also a brand out there called Charra's that makes baked corn tostada shells with no oil. I like to break some of them up and dip in a super-fresh salsa.
- Freeze-dried fruits and veggies are super-tasty, low-fat snacking options that help you stay on track. And now more than ever, companies have options for you to enjoy plant-strong snacks on the go (just be sure to read labels, as brands change ingredients and formulas all the time).
- Bare makes a whole line of different options. Read the labels carefully here, though, because many of them have fatty ingredients. But their apple chips (they have a few varieties) are especially good.
- Another company called Barnana makes really cool chewy organic banana snacks that have zero fat and are really satisfying. Avoid the coconut, peanut butter, chocolate, or coffee flavors, though, as they are all 30 to 50 percent fat. Focus on the one that is only bananas.

- Karen's Naturals has a line of freeze-dried peaches, blueberries, strawberries, mangos, and even veggies that are really great to have on hand.

Finally, you can always go the dried fruit route—apricots, dates, figs, and so on. Find out what you like, but any of these options can be very satiating without taking in a high-fat snack food.

Keep in mind, these are satisfying because they have sugars but all naturally occurring sugars, not junky added sugars. The ones out there that are 100 percent fruit are OK. Even Kind bars are getting in on the act and offer 100 percent pure fruit bars.

SUGAR AND SALT

Adding some sugar or salt to any meal is totally fine. Don't go crazy, but don't worry about it either. If it helps you to eat your starch and enjoy it, that's fine.

COOKING WITHOUT OIL

Some people might find the concept of cooking without oil confusing. You may be accustomed to using oil for stir-fries or to sauté foods. You're done with that. Get a good nonstick pan or skillet and use veggie broth, a fruit or veggie juice, or just water to sauté. Try just about any liquids other than oils, and make sure you have enough in the pan. Liquids evaporate quicker than oil so don't be afraid to use more. You'll find you can make tasty stir-fries with some low-sodium tamari or soy sauce or just water. Some people cook with wine or even beer. While we discourage alcohol while you're stopping your acne, it can be done; as long as you keep enough liquid in the pan, your food will cook fine.

BATCH COOKING

Ensuring success means thinking in advance about your meals. Some people take one day a week (sometimes two) and make everything they're going to eat the rest of the week. To do that, just make your food in bulk. This works especially well with soups, sauces, stews, chili, and grains. You can make large quantities and put them in airtight, sealed containers, and freeze them. Put a label with the date on the container for future reference. Then you can use these foods throughout the week. Remember that tomorrow's leftovers came from tonight's dinner. The clear skin scout's motto is be prepared.

Foods that can be easily made in bulk include:

1. Baked potatoes, mashed potatoes, sweet potatoes
2. Brown rice, barley, pasta, and other grains
3. Stews, chili, soups
4. Beans, peas, lentils
5. Burritos, veggie burgers, lasagna

TIPS FOR STORING FOODS

Our favorite food storage containers are plain old Pyrex stacking bowls. They come with lids and are great for storing large batches in the fridge or freezer. They're also handy for reheating in the microwave. They are not very expensive and are readily available at outlets like Amazon.com, Target, Walmart, Bed Bath & Beyond, and many other stores.

ACNE ADVICE:
From Rip Esselstyn

I've had the pleasure of knowing the Nelson family since Nina and Randa were little kids. The last time I was at their house, I was really impressed with how they had three Instant Pot pressure cookers going at all times of day. One had steel-cut oats, one had pinto beans, and one had brown rice. At any point in the day, they'd take a spoonful of rice and beans or have some oatmeal and layer some banana or veggies on top. There was *always* a selection of plant-strong goodness ready to eat!

You might not need that kind of system in your home, but it really all does start with a system. Having a few Crock-Pot slow cookers or Instant Pots going with grains, beans, potatoes, and/or oats is a great way to quickly assemble delicious, plant-strong meals at the drop of a hat. But depending on your situation, it might work out better for you to pick up a bunch of frozen, precooked grains like quinoa and rice, or some frozen fruits and veggies. Fresh, precut, and washed veggies work great too, plus some varieties of no-salt-added canned beans. This system has worked wonders for more than twenty thousand people who have participated in our Engine 2 Seven-Day Rescue Challenge that follows the same protocol as this book. You'll have all the ingredients you need to assemble a delicious snack or meal in minutes, whether it's after work, after school, or on the weekend.

USEFUL KITCHEN TOOLS

There are a few kitchen tools we use just about every day because they make healthy eating so easy. We tend to eat a lot of rice, potatoes, oatmeal, beans, lentils, and so on, in a variety of combinations. Here are some of the gadgets and tools we like.

PRESSURE COOKER

Pressure cooking is the process of cooking food using water (or another cooking liquid) in a sealed pot known as a pressure cooker. Pressure cookers trap steam while the food is cooking, which increases the temperature so that food cooks faster. The higher temperature also forces liquid into the food and keeps it moist and tender. The higher the pressure, the faster things cook, and the shorter the cooking time.

It used to be that a pressure cooker required a certain amount of attention and work. You would put it on the stove, warm it up, add foods, add liquids, cover it, bring it up to pressure, then turn the heat down, monitor it, remove it at the right moment, and so forth. It wasn't that hard but it was a little involved and required paying close attention so the food came out right. Today, that's all changed. Electric pressure cookers came along, and basically you put the water and food in, put on the lid, press a button, and walk away. The cooker does the rest, and a short time later, you have perfect food every time.

An electric pressure cooker that we recommend is called the Instant Pot. As Rip noticed, we actually have three of these out at all times on our kitchen counter: we may have rice or potatoes in one, legumes or soup in another, steamed veggies in the third. The stove rarely gets a workout because it's so quick and easy to just dump something in a pot, press a button, and go about your business knowing that you'll have a healthy meal ready for you in just a few minutes. Having one pressure cooker is great, but more is better. They can cook things quickly, and they're so easy to operate. Everyone in our family can use it. Just measure out the rice (or potatoes or oatmeal or beans or whatever you want to cook), pour in a specified amount of water, put the lid on and lock it, press a button, and that's it. Walk away, the pot does the rest, including bringing it to pressure, and when it's done, bringing pressure down and keeping the food warm. In the morning we might put rice in one cooker and beans in the other, press a button, and in anywhere from ten to twenty-five minutes (depending on what kind of rice) the rice will be ready. The beans may take up to eighty minutes but with no one having to pay attention. We then have a nice supply of delicious food for the rest of the day, or maybe for a few days depending on how much we make.

A pressure cooker allows you to steam veggies conveniently and quickly, make large batches of steel cut oatmeal, whole grains like quinoa, barley, and rice, cook beans quickly without a need to presoak them, steam veggies—you name it! You can make soups, stews, and chili, and it cooks them in a more intense way so that the flavors are more concentrated.

And to repeat, the best thing is you can "set it and forget it": most electric pressure cookers can be programmed and will automatically switch to "warm" mode once done. You can leave and come back hours later, and your food will still be ready and not overcooked. Many pressure cookers have a timer function, so you can set it to make your oatmeal thirty minutes before you wake up, or to have dinner ready and waiting when you get home. Instant Pot even came out with a small, six-quart version that's about eighty dollars, perfect for a student in a dorm or for traveling. (And we don't have any financial relationship with the company; we just think they're terrific. There are other brands of electric pressure cookers that are probably useful, too.)

BLENDER

Great for making soups, smoothies, fruit soft serve, spreads, you name it.

FOOD PROCESSOR

If you've used a food processor before, you know it can be used to chop, shred, slice, or julienne large quantities of veggies, to purée sauces and spreads, and to make sorbet and dough, as well as many other uses. In our house, we actually don't use ours all that often, preferring the blender, chopper, or mini food processor for most jobs.

CHOPPER OR MINI FOOD PROCESSOR

There are a variety of smaller choppers and mincers that are great for taking the work out of slicing and dicing veggies. You lay a vegetable across a grid and then press down on a top piece that cuts the veggie to the desired size and style, depending on which grate you select. Mini food processors, with a three- to four-cup capacity, can rapidly process small amounts of food.

ACNE ADVICE:
From Chef AJ

For making something quickly when you get home, I recommend an air fryer. You can take a potato or sweet potato and make the most amazing crisp and delicious french fries in twenty minutes without any oil. If you have already batch-cooked some potatoes, it will take even less time.

RICE COOKER

This isn't necessary if you have a pressure cooker, but it's nice to have on hand to make rice.

CITRUS SQUEEZER

As the name says, this device squeezes juice from citrus fruits.

SET OF GLASS BOWLS OR TUPPERWARE

Good for storing leftovers or for storing batch meals.

ACNE ADVICE:
From Chef AJ

To make satisfying desserts, you can use pitted dates in place of sugar and oats instead of nuts or flour. Believe it or not, frozen fruit makes a delicious dessert. When you freeze grapes or cherries, they taste amazing. And with ripe bananas, you can even make sorbet by using a Vitamix, a food processor, or a Yonanas machine. Top with fresh fruit like berries for a delicious sundae!

YONANAS MACHINE

This is a fun, relatively inexpensive kitchen appliance that uses 100 percent frozen fruit to make cheap, healthy soft-serve ice cream and desserts. Making delicious ice cream is easy: freeze a bunch of ripe bananas (after removing the skin) and press them through the Yonanas machine. You will swear what results is delicious ice cream! Add a little maple syrup or fat-free cocoa and it's pure heaven.

PANINI GRILL PRESS

There are multiple fun things you can make with a panini press, but our favorite panini-press specials are veggie burgers. You can sear your homemade burgers perfectly on both sides, and it's much easier to get the perfect burger with this press than a frying pan. Toss some onions on the grill while you're grilling your burger, and you are well on your way to a fantastic meal.

ACNE ADVICE:
From Mary McDougall

Acceptable materials for cookware include glass, stainless steel, iron, non-stick coated pans, and bake ware (such as DuPont's SilverStone, Teflon, or Farberware Millennium), silicone-coated bakeware (such as Baker's Secret), and porcelain. Nonstick cookware makes it easy to avoid fats and oil. Pots and pans can be a significant source of minerals and other metals. Small amounts of minerals are essential; however, large amounts of iron, magnesium, and zinc can increase your risk of heart disease. We recommend that you avoid using aluminum cookware because of an association with Alzheimer's disease.

STEAMER BASKET

If you have a pressure cooker, they generally come with a basket for steaming foods, but if not, consider getting a steamer basket. It's usually made out of stainless steel and goes inside a pot. It has legs that keep the food in the basket above the boiling water and allow the steam to cook the veggies.

OTHER USEFUL TOOLS

Cutting boards
Garlic press
Good set of kitchen knives
Measuring cups

Nonstick frying pans
Salad tongs
Set of pots for boiling
Soup ladle

ACNE ADVICE:
From Neal Barnard, MD

Need dinner now? Try easy pita pizzas. Slather whole wheat pita bread with no-oil pizza sauce and load up on veggie toppings. Think onions, peppers, sundried tomatoes, and artichokes. Sprinkle with oregano and bake at 350 degrees for seven to eight minutes. Faster than delivery!

PLAN TO WIN

Remember to start a food journal when you begin the Clear Skin Diet to keep track in case you need to analyze and tweak your eating. We also would like to suggest that you explore books by experts like those we list in the Resources section, visit their websites, or watch their YouTube channels. By increasing your knowledge about plant-based diets, you will reinforce your determination to succeed and find even more encouragement.

11

THE CLEAR SKIN PANTRY

by Nina

A very effective way to ensure your long-term success on the Clear Skin Diet is to clean out your kitchen. And I'm not talking about wiping down the counters and scrubbing the floor, Cinderella. If possible, dispose of the foods you're no longer going to eat. Bag them up and put them in a Dumpster so they're nowhere near your house to seduce you. And no, don't give it away; just get rid of it. If you don't want to eat it anymore because it's not good for you, do you really want to inflict that on someone else? But in any event, just be rid of it. Get it out of your consciousness by getting it out of your house. It's much easier to control your environment than to try to control willpower. Eliminate temptations. Make sure your home, car, school, and work are safe places by keeping plenty of the most healthful food choices around at all times. Then you don't have to work on yourself when it comes to better eating. The problem isn't you; it's the food we're all surrounded by.

ACNE ADVICE:
From Chef AJ

Staying out of the Pleasure Trap is hard because we weren't designed for the environment we are living in. Unhealthy food is cheap and ubiquitous, and the only environment you can control is your own home. The number-one rule for healthy living is no junk food in the home. We have to work harder on our environment than we do ourselves. I like to say, "If it's in your house, it's in your mouth!" And it's not a question of *if* you will eat it, only *when*!

The easiest way to deal with temptation is to avoid it. High-calorie foods are incredibly tempting. We are biologically wired to use the least effort to seek out the highest calorie foods. Our DNA is hardwired to reward us when we eat very rich food. That's why rich food gives us the most pleasure. In an environment of scarcity, such as where our species lived for millions of years, being driven and rewarded by our biology to eat high-calorie foods whenever possible was a very useful survival trait. But today, when we're surrounded by processed high-calorie foods on every corner, it's deadly. If you have bad food lurking in your fridge, it's going to be waiting for you when you're hungry, tempting you, calling your name, trying to lure you back into your former habits. But you can't eat what's not in your home, so this is why your first step in creating a clear skin pantry is to clear your cabinets, fridge, and freezer of foods containing animal products, oil, processed foods, and overt fats.

Now you can have fun restocking your kitchen with the kind of healthy foods you're going to be enjoying from now on, foods to heal your acne.

Next, get to know your local grocery store so it's easy for you to shop for the foods you will be eating. And put effort into keeping your pantry well stocked with the recommended foods. Having healthy foods around whenever you're hungry will keep you happy—and out of trouble.

SHOP FOR THESE CLEAR SKIN DIET FOODS

You will need to purchase fresh produce generally at least once a week, but most of the bulk and convenience foods we're recommending have fairly long shelf lives. Frozen, precut, and canned foods can save you time and provide ease in meal preparation. Choosing foods that are quick and easy is a big help, and they're just as nutritious.

CONVENIENCE ITEMS

Although you want to get as much of your food in its fresh, "as grown in the ground" form, here are some packaged goods that are super excellent and convenient.

Frozen fruits and vegetables. Frozen fruits and veggies can be your best allies. You can always whip out a bag of frozen berries and add them to a hot bowl of oatmeal, or microwave a bag of frozen veggie blend to add to some beans, rice, or potatoes. They are also excellent additions to any soup, stew, or entrée and can even be served as a quick side dish.

Precut vegetables and prepared lettuce. These are available in most produce departments nationwide and can simplify vegetable preparation for meals and snacks.

Canned fruit. Look for those that are either packed in juice or water. These can be used for desserts or snacks.

Canned and/or dehydrated soups (low fat and no oil). These are convenient for quick lunches and dinners or meals on the road. They can be an appetizer, a main course, or as a sauce over your starch. Twenty years ago, Dr. McDougall started a line of food products called Right Foods, to make it easier for people to follow the McDougall Program. Right Foods has a variety of soups that are perfect for when you're traveling or in a hurry.

Packaged pasta or marinara sauces. Always get fat-free (low-sodium when possible) pasta sauces: add additional vegetables such as onions, mushrooms, and garlic to create a quick sauce to use over pasta, rice, or potatoes.

Canned or dried beans and legumes. Legumes are a great source of fiber, protein, and many nutrients and are very affordable. Eating them regularly decreases the risk of many diseases and helps maintain a healthy weight. Having a variety available is useful. When buying in cans, try to get the no-salt-added variety. Among the many canned beans and legumes available are pinto beans, black beans, kidney beans, butter beans, cannellini beans, garbanzo beans, lentils, split peas, black-eyes peas, and red beans.

Canned tomatoes. When getting canned foods of any kind—not just tomatoes—we generally try to find low-salt or no-salt versions. That's the healthiest way to eat—lower sodium. However for the purposes of the Clear Skin Diet and getting rid of your acne, sodium is not really a factor, so you don't need to freak out about salt to lose your acne.

Veggie stock. You can find a variety of low-sodium, oil-free vegetable stocks and broths in aseptic boxes or cans.

Fat-free plant milks. Use plant-based milks for your cereal or for recipes calling for milk substitutes. Make sure the plant milk fat-free; we don't know of any nut milks that are fat-free. In the Recipes section, we have recipes for oat milk and banana milk, which we recommend over any store-bought plant milks.

Frozen pizza dough. We recommend Kabuli brand, an oil-free whole grain pizza crust. Just add pasta sauce, veggies, and bake. We also recommend Engine 2 Plant-Strong Stone Baked Pizza Crusts, available at Whole Foods Markets, which are oil-free and whole grain.

Various frozen veggie mixes. You can buy a variety of veggie mixes, for example Italian Blend (Jennifer's Garden), Mediterranean Blend (Green Giant), or California Blend (Birds Eye).

Hash browns. Packaged hash browns sold in the frozen section are great as a stand-alone breakfast or for adding to casseroles or tacos.

Sorbet. This is a healthy dessert if you're looking for something cold and sweet. Sorbets may contain a lot of sugar, but they're dairy-free. When it's hot out, these decadent-tasting (but with no decadent ingredients) desserts are super cool.

WHOLE GRAINS

Grains are derived from the seeds of grasses and are inherently nutritious. They have no cholesterol and are low fat and high fiber. Thousands of published studies confirm the healthful benefits of whole grains. (It's worth noting that the cereal industry paid for most of those studies, so take them with a "whole grain" of salt!)

Brown rice. Great for heart health and weight management; an anti-inflammatory, satisfying starch.

Corn tortillas. High fiber, rich in vitamins and minerals, oil-free, and lower in calories than flour tortillas.

Couscous. Rich in fiber, good source of protein.

Crackers. Whole grain and baked, no oil.

Dry cereal. Shredded Wheat, puffed grains (corn, rice, millet, wheat), Grape-Nuts, Cheerios, Oatios, Erewhon Crispy Brown Rice cereal, or any cereal that contains a whole grain and no other added ingredients (for example, Grape-Nuts contains only wheat). Eat with banana milk or homemade oat milk.

Multigrain hot cereal. Make sure the ingredients list "whole wheat" or "whole grain" rather than just "wheat cereal."

Popcorn (microwavable, oil free, salt free). Healthy snack as long as you keep the oils and high-fat sauces off.

Quinoa. Protein-rich, very high fiber source of omega-3 fats.

Rolled oats. Rich in fiber, protein rich, heart healthy.

Whole grain bagels. Better choice than plain or "white" bagels or bread.

Whole grain bread. Packed with nutrients, shown to reduce heart disease, type 2 diabetes, obesity, and some cancers; Food for Life brand makes a variety of super-healthy whole grain breads. And let's be real: bread is life.

Whole grain flours. Just make sure it says "whole grain" on the package.

Whole grain pancake or muffin mixes. You just add water or a plant milk, and you're ready to cook.

Whole grain pasta. Brown rice pasta, whole wheat pasta, buckwheat pasta—high in minerals and B vitamins.

Whole wheat pita bread. Good fiber and protein source.

Whole wheat tortillas. Nutrient-packed, make great wraps.

SNACKS, SAUCES, SWEETENERS, SPICES

Jams and jellies. Look for the least processed, like fruit spreads made of fruits as well as low-sugar jams.

Dried fruits. There are lots of delicious dried fruits: dates, figs, raisins, apricots, bananas, berries; just avoid them if they have added sugar or oil.

Syrups. Brown rice syrup and maple syrup.

Sauces and condiments. These can give your meal just the kick it needs to take it to the next level. Use them for stir-fries or with a starch and veggies: ketchup, hoisin sauce, ginger stir-fry sauces, curry sauces, fat-free mushroom sauce, oil-free teriyaki sauce, barbecue sauces, Cajun sauces, unsweetened applesauce, mustard, Tabasco sauce, hot sauces, vegetarian Worcestershire sauce, steak sauce, balsamic vinegar, red wine vinegar, rice vinegar, brown rice vinegar, and oil-free salad dressings.

Baking powder and baking soda. Great for baking and making pancakes and used in a variety of recipes.

Seasonings and spices. As you reduce or eliminate added salt, sugar, and oil in your diet, you will begin to appreciate the wonderful natural flavors of food. But you may still want a little "spice" in your life. Fortunately, there are many salt-free spices, seasonings, and blends available. If something tastes bland, lemon juice, spices, or garlic can turn it around. There are premixed blends of salt-free Italian, Mexican, Indian, southern, and many other varieties available, such as jambalaya spice mix or Mrs. Dash seasoning blends. Other spices and herbs that can provide flavor include ground cinnamon, ground black pepper, garlic powder, chili power, dried dillweed, onion powder, ground turmeric, ground cumin, curry powder, oregano, basil, marjoram, and dried parsley. Try adding iodized salt, low-sodium soy sauce, Bragg Liquid Aminos, chili paste, cornstarch, vanilla extract (alcohol-free), or sweet pickle relish to spark up a dish.

Salsa. Salsa is a fantastic condiment for many occasions and foods. And it's salsa! Need I say more? Who in their right mind doesn't like salsa.

Nutritional yeast. Yeast is a perfect addition to any meal; it provides nutrition but is low in calories and is great for making creamy sauces in place of cheese or dairy. We scoop this stuff onto everything.

FRESH FRUITS AND VEGGIES

Fruits. Whichever are your favorites, mix it up: apples, bananas, berries, grapefruit, grapes, lemons, limes, melons (cantaloupe, watermelon, honeydew, etc.), mango, nectarines, oranges or tangerines, papaya, peaches, pears, plums.

Veggies. Broccoli, bell peppers (different colors and varieties), cauliflower, carrots, celery, cilantro, collard greens, cucumbers, kale (any type), garlic, ginger root, green onions, mixed salad greens, mushrooms (crimini, portobello, shiitake, etc.), onions, parsley, potatoes (russet, sweet, Yukon Gold, etc.), spinach, tomatoes, zucchini.

SHOPPING LIST SUMMARY

Go to the supermarket prepared. Think about what you want to eat in the week ahead; refer to the list in this chapter of recommended foods or use the summary list below.

Beans and Other Canned Foods (no added salt, if possible)

Black beans

Canned artichoke hearts in water

Canned chopped green chiles

Canned tomatoes

Cannellini beans

Garbanzo beans

Kidney beans

Pinto beans

Whole Grains and Breads

Brown rice

Corn tortillas

Couscous

Dry cereal (Shredded Wheat, puffed corn, rice, millet, or wheat, Grape-Nuts,

Cheerios, Oatios, Erewhon Crispy Brown Rice cereal)

Multigrain hot cereal

Oats (rolled, steel-cut)

Popcorn (microwavable, oil-free, salt-free)

Quinoa
Whole grain bagels
Whole grain bread

Whole grain pasta
Whole wheat pita bread
Whole wheat tortillas

Frozen Items

Frozen mixed berries
Frozen pizza dough (Kabuli)
Frozen veggies (assorted

mixed veggies, pepper and
onion mix, corn kernels,
lima beans)

Herbs, Spices, and Seasonings (ideally all spices should be salt-free)

Basil
Chili powder
Curry powder
Dried dillweed
Dried parsley
Garlic powder (salt-free)
Ground black pepper
Ground cinnamon
Ground cumin

Iodized salt
Italian seasoning blend
Jambalaya spice mix
Marjoram
Mrs. Dash seasoning blends
Onion powder
Oregano
Turmeric

Sauces and Other

Applesauce (unsweetened)
Balsamic vinegar
Chili paste (*sambal oelek* or
    other)
Cocoa powder (unsweetened)
Cornstarch
Ketchup
Maple syrup
Mustard
Nutritional yeast flakes
Pasta sauce (fat- and oil-free)

Red pepper sauce (Tabasco or
    other)
Rice vinegar (unseasoned)
Salsa
Soy sauce or tamari
    (low-sodium)
Sweet pickle relish
Vanilla extract (alcohol-free)
Vegetable broth (we prefer
    Pacific Low Sodium
    Vegetable Broth)

Fresh and Dried Fruit

Apples
Bananas
Berries (any type)
Dates
Grapefruit
Grapes
Lemons
Limes
Mango

Melons (cantaloupe, water-
    melons, honeydew, etc.)
Nectarines
Oranges or tangerines
Papaya
Peaches
Pears
Plums
Raisins (make sure no added
    oil)

Fresh Veggies

Bell peppers (any color or
    variety)
Broccoli
Carrots
Cauliflower
Celery
Cilantro
Collard greens
Cucumbers
Garlic
Ginger root, fresh
Green onions

Kale (any type)
Mixed salad greens
Mushrooms (crimini, porto-
    bello, shiitake, etc.)
Onions
Parsley
Potatoes (russet, sweet pota-
    toes, Yukon Gold, etc.)
Spinach
Squash (any type)
Tomatoes
Zucchini

ACNE ADVICE:
From Ann Esselstyn

Once you understand the damage oil, meat, and dairy do, it isn't so hard to avoid them. In buying packaged food, the trick is to read ingredients. Always. Never believe what the front of the package says. Read the ingredients! Lurking in a can of tomatoes and basil could be olive oil, or buttermilk and coconut in a package of crackers. When you see those ingredients and know what harm they can do, it is easy to avoid them.

READING FOOD LABELS

The best foods for your skin—and your health in general—are the ones that don't come with a label: whole plant foods are skin friendly: fruits, veggies, legumes, and whole grains. You want to do your best to limit packaged and processed foods. That said, there will be times when—because you're in a hurry or a recipe calls for it or you are dying to try something different—you're going to buy processed foods. And (gasp) that's when you need to pay attention to food labels.

    Registered dietitian Jeff Novick, MS, RD, is the person who taught us about understanding the complicated world of food labels. Jeff ran the Pritikin Longevity Center in South Florida for many years, and for more than a decade he has been working with John McDougall, MD, at the McDougall Health Clinic in Santa Rosa, California. He is also a trained chef, so he really knows how to make healthy taste GOOD. Jeff's teachings about nutrition are virtually the gospel of healthy eating. Randa and I are so grateful to have known Jeff since we were eight years old and to have had the privilege of working with him on an amazing four-part video series called *Jeff Novick's Fast Food*. (See the Resources section at the end of this book for how to find Jeff and his excellent work.) Chef Jeff helped teach us how to cook!

Jeff has spent decades researching and coming up with a straightforward, easy strategy for reading those confusing food labels. Learn his principles and you'll understand what you might be eating. The rest of this chapter is based on Jeff's work.

FOOD LABELS ARE MISLEADING

The first thing to learn about label reading is that you can't believe any claim that's found on the front of a package. Food manufacturers inflate positive nutritional claims while minimizing the negative. They get away with this because there are no global standards to standardize the labeling of packaged food. Why are labeling laws so lax and nutrition data information baffling? Let's just say the confusion in understanding food labels benefits the food companies, not the consumer.

What do you want to find out when reading a food label? Two basic things are important for you to know on the Clear Skin Diet: (1) the ingredients, and (2) the percentage of calories that come from fat. We're also going to give you a guideline for sodium, but that's not critical for acne.

THE INGREDIENTS

The first thing you examine when you are evaluating a food is the list of ingredients. What are the ingredients? Are there several of them? Fewer is always better than more. Are there long words you can't pronounce? That's usually a bad sign. Ideally, you want to see a simple, short list of plant ingredients. And since you're eating the starch-based Clear Skin Diet, you should be looking for complex carbs, not refined ones. That means you want to see words describing grains like *whole, stone ground, rolled, cracked,* and *sprouted*. These are words expressly approved by the FDA to only describe whole foods. Brown rice is also a whole food, and wheat berries and bulgur are intact grains. So look for ingredients like whole grain flour, rolled oats, cracked wheat, and stone-ground corn.

You want to try to avoid refined carbohydrates, which can't use those words. Refined carbs may have deceptive adjectives like wheat, white, durum, semolina, bleached, and unbleached. Be aware of words like *enriched* and *fortified*. All these words apply to processed foods. (Foods only need to be enriched and fortified when most of their nutrition has been stripped out of them.)

Of course you don't want to see animal products in the ingredients list or any oils. We are consuming foods low in fats, so *avoid* any foods that list:

❖ anything containing meat, chicken, fish, turkey, eggs, dairy, cheese, butter, sour cream, yogurt, whipped cream, ice cream, lard, whey, or casein (animal fats)

❖ any oil-based fats like olive oil (or any oil), or saturated vegetable fats like cocoa butter and coconut, palm, and palm kernel oil

❖ any hydrogenated or partially hydrogenated (trans-fat) vegetable oils, margarine, or shortening (man-made saturated fats)

You're also going to avoid specific plant-based fats that the Clear Skin Diet excludes. Ingredients should not contain any of the following:

❖ Avocados

❖ Nuts, seeds, or nut butters (like peanut butter or PB2 powdered peanut butter)

❖ Soy or soymilk

❖ Hummus

❖ Coconut

❖ Olives

If you're considering a product that doesn't contain any of these ingredients, it's probably a plant-based, very low fat food, and that's exactly what you want. When embarking on the Clear Skin Diet, ideally any processed foods you *do* eat will be very low in fat or fat-free. Eating whole foods is always going to be better for healing acne than processed foods.

THE PERCENTAGE OF CALORIES FROM FAT IN THE FOOD

Let's say your acne is reduced and you think you might want to add some additional processed foods back into your diet, aim for *no more than 10 to 15 percent of calories from fat*, and see how that impacts your acne.

How do you calculate the percentage of fat in a food? You can do it with the (confusing) information provided on food labels. First, find the number of calories in the serving. Then find the number of calories from fat. Then divide the number of calories from fat into the total calories of a serving.

Let's say a label looks like this:

The label shows that one serving is 260 calories, and that serving contains 120 calories from fat. If we divide 120 (calories from fat) by 260 (total calories) we get .46. That means this product is 46 percent fat. That's a lot of fat and way beyond the 10 to 15 percent of calories from fat we're shooting for. This item would be a NO in terms of fat content.

Here's another example.

This shows that a serving of this food contains 32 calories from fat, out of 222 total calories. If we take 32 calories and divide it by 222, we get .14. So this food is 14 percent calories from fat, and we could go with this one as it's at the upper end of our limit of no more than 10 to 15 percent calories from fat. This food is OK—based on fat content. Of course, you have to look at the ingredients list to be sure.

Another way to calculate the percentage of fat calories is to multiply the total number of calories per serving by .1. When you multiply total calories by .1, that will tell you how many calories equals 10 percent of total calories. Then you compare that number to the number of calories from fat listed on the label to see whether it's in the right range or too high.

For example, the label at the top of the following page shows a total of 200 calories.

Nutrition Facts
Serving Size 172 g

Amount Per Serving

Calories 200			Calories from Fat 8
			% Daily Value*
Total Fat 1g			1%
Saturated Fat 0g			1%
Trans Fat			
Cholesterol 0mg			0%
Sodium 7mg			0%
Total Carbohydrate 36g			12%
Dietary Fiber 11g			45%
Sugars 6g			
Protein 13g			
Vitamin A	1%	Vitamin C	1%
Calcium	4%	Iron	24%

*Percent Daily Values are based on a 2,000 calorie diet. Your daily values may be higher or lower depending on your calorie needs.

Nutrition Facts
Serving Size 1 cup 185g (185 g)

Amount Per Serving

Calories 222			Calories from Fat 32
			% Daily Value*
Total Fat 4g			5%
Saturated Fat			5%
Trans Fat			
Cholesterol 0mg			0%
Sodium 13mg			1%
Total Carbohydrate 39g			13%
Dietary Fiber 5g			21%
Sugars			
Protein 8g			
Vitamin A	0%	Vitamin C	0%
Calcium	3%	Iron	15%

*Percent Daily Values are based on a 2,000 calorie diet. Your daily values may be higher or lower depending on your calorie needs:

	Calories	2,000	2,500
Total Fat	Less than	65g	80g
Sat Fat	Less than	20g	25g
Cholesterol	Less than	300mg	300mg
Sodium	Less than	2,400mg	2,400mg
Total Carbihydrate		300g	375g
Fiber		25g	30g

If you multiply that by .1 you get 20 calories. So that means 10 percent of calories from fat of 200 calories is 20 calories. Now look at the label and see whether the calories from fat is 20 or fewer. In fact, it's showing only 8 calories from fat, so this is well below the 20 calories that represent acceptable level in terms of fat of 10 percent of calories from fat.

Now if you are outside the United States, labels are different and will show the total calories and the total grams in fat per serving. To calculate the total number of calories of fat per serving, you must first multiply the total grams of fat per serving by 10, before running the rest of the calculation.

Here is an example of a food label in the European Union:

Total calories for this 100-gram serving is 117 (kcal is the same as calories). The fat is listed as 8 grams. We multiply that 8 grams times 10 and get 80 calories.

Now we run the percentage of fat calculation as before: 80 calories (of fat) divided by 117 (total) calories, which is .68, or 68 percent of calories are from fat in this product. This is a very fatty product and is nowhere near the 10 to 15 percent calories of fat we're looking for. But of course, if you look at the ingredients list on the label, you'll see it contains milk, as well as nuts, both of which are not part of the Clear Skin Diet. This fails on both ingredients as well as how much fat it contains. (This method for European labels has you multiple fat grams times 10, but actually a gram of fat contains 9 calories. We round it up to 10 to make the math easier, but if you were trying to be completely accurate, you would multiply by 9. But it's not necessary to be that precise.)

Nutrition Facts
Serving Size 172 g

Amount Per Serving		
Calories 200		Calories from Fat 8
		% Daily Value*
Total Fat 1g		1%
Saturated Fat 0g		1%
Trans Fat		
Cholesterol 0mg		0%
Sodium 7mg		0%
Total Carbohydrate 36g		12%
Dietary Fiber 11g		45%
Sugars 6g		
Protein 13g		
Vitamin A	1%	Vitamin C	1%
Calcium	4%	Iron	24%

*Percent Daily Values are based on a 2,000 calorie diet. Your daily values may be higher or lower depending on your calorie needs.

Nutrition Facts

	Per 100 g
Energy	485 kJ / 117 kcal
Fat	8 g
Of which Saturates	3.7 g
Carbohydrate	9 g
Of which Sugars	8 g
Protein	1.4 g
Salt	0.02 g
Vitamin C	14,81 mg 19% RI*

Salt content is exclusively due to the presence of naturally occuring sodium.

*Reference intake of an average adult (8 400 kJ / 2 000 kcal)

INGREDIENTS: Mandarin Oranges (37.9%), Light Whipping Cream (Milk), Pears (12.4%), Peaches (7.7%), Banana (5.9%), English Walnuts (Tree Nuts)

HOMEMADE PLANT MILKS

Generally, we don't recommend store-bought plant milks, other than rice milk, because of the higher fat content than homemade plant milks. You can find homemade plant milks in the Recipes section. Here is a list of common plant milks sold in supermarkets and the average amount of fat each contains, from lowest to highest:

Rice milk: 16 percent calories from fat
Oat milk: 27 percent calories from fat
Hemp milk: 32 percent calories from fat
Soy milk: 36 percent calories from fat
Almond milk: 50 percent calories from fat
Coconut milk: 88 percent calories from fat

Some participants who cleared their skin the fastest said they avoided plant milks altogether, initially. Homemade plant milks tend to be a little less processed and lower in fat than store-bought. But again, if you are using plant milks but having trouble clearing your acne, try skipping them and perhaps substituting water, applesauce, or banana milk—until your acne clears.

WHAT DOES A CHOCOLATE LABEL REVEAL?

Can you tell from a chocolate nutrition information label whether or not it would promote acne? In chapter 3 we discussed Dr. Fulton's 1969 acne-chocolate study—the problematic one paid for by the Chocolate Manufacturers of America that purported to show chocolate doesn't cause acne. It turns out, Dr. Fulton did not get the last word.

In 2015, dermatologists at Chulalongkorn University in Bangkok, Thailand, decided to do their own acne-chocolate study. The researchers noted that dermatologists have long followed the "old dermatology maxim...that chocolate and food in general are not related to acne exacerbation." But, the researchers continued, there is increasingly compelling scientific evidence making it clear that certain foods actually do promote acne.

To test whether chocolate causes acne, the researchers enrolled twenty-five acne-prone male subjects who were asked to consume 25 grams of 99 percent dark chocolate daily for four weeks. Dark chocolate was selected because it does not contain dairy and thus, the researchers wrote, the well-documented

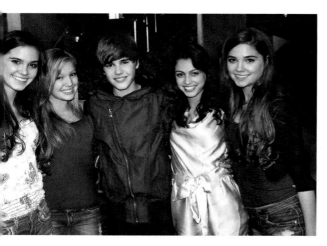

On "U Smile" set
with Justin Bieber

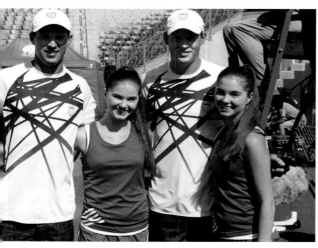

ESPIN "Doublemint
Twins" commercial
with Bryan twins

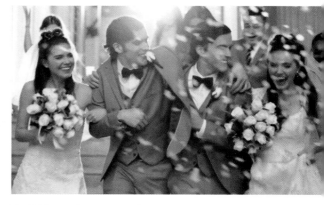

BMW "Twins" commercial

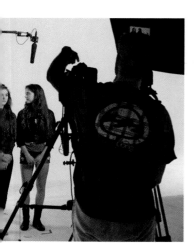

Nintendo commercial

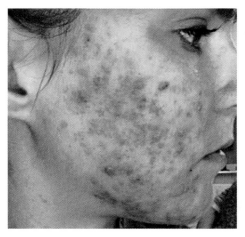

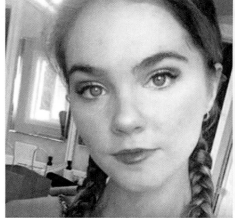

Nina after 6 weeks on diet

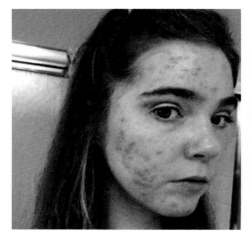

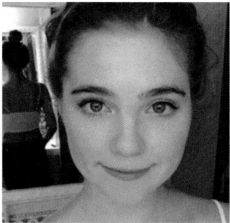

Randa after 6 weeks on diet

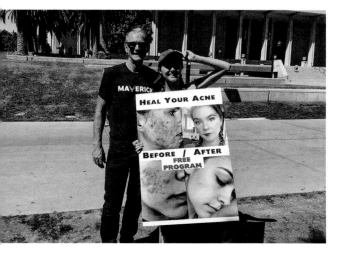

Nina and Dad recruit
study participants

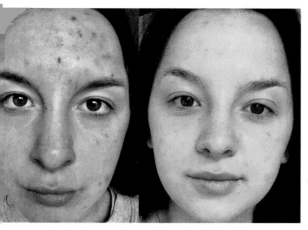

Kendall Boyrs-
progress in 11 days on diet

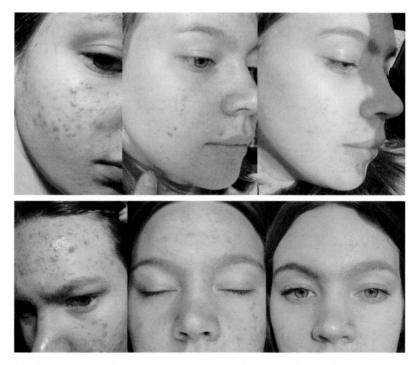

Monica Marcinkiewicz-progress in 14 days and four months on diet

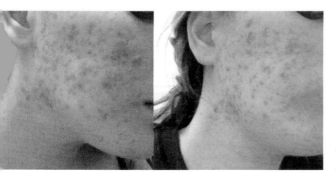

Olivia right cheek
after 14 days on diet

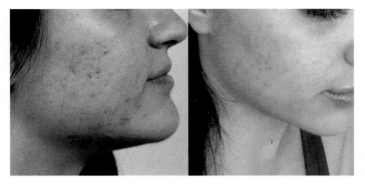

Francesca's PIH fades
after 7 weeks on diet

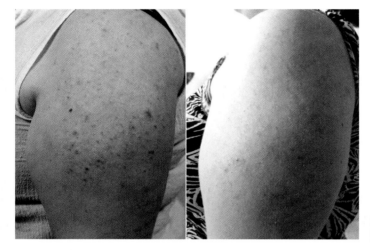

Maria DiGrazia cleared
her arm acne in 6 weeks

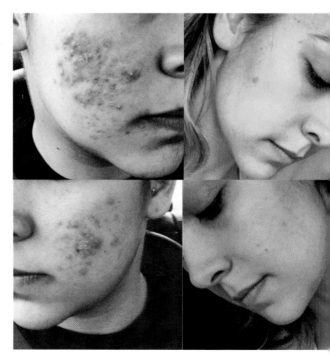

Kira's acne faded
quickly on the diet

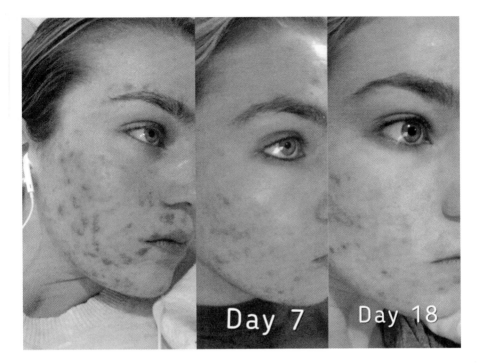

Day 7   Day 18

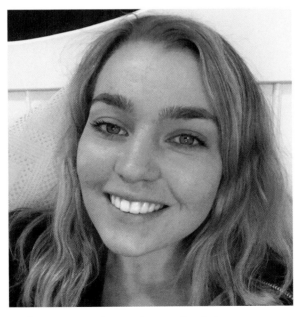

Ashley's success after 25 days on the diet

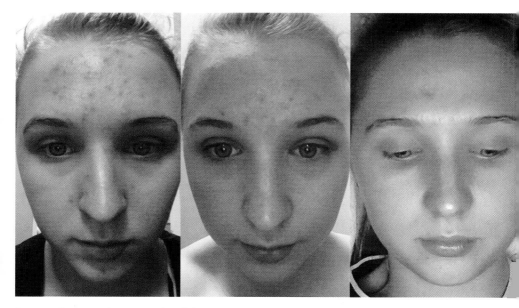

Dani on day 10 and two months of diet

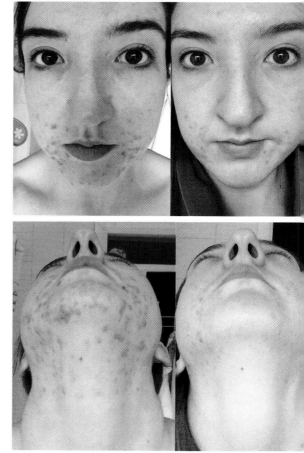

Robyn after 60 days on diet

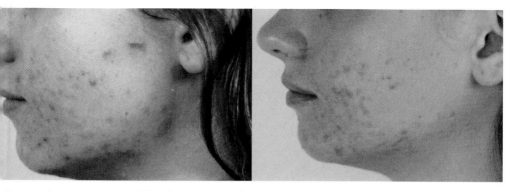

yl's acne fades on 30 days, PIH takes longer to clear

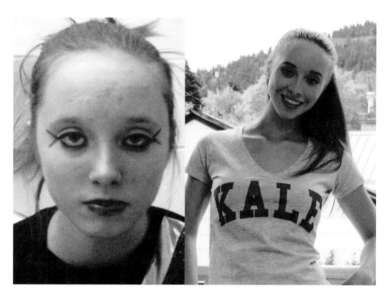

Kara's acne vanished and she got fit

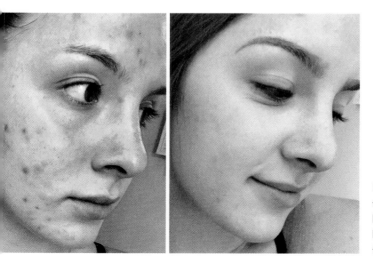

Kendall Boyrs went off the Clear Skin Diet and broke out, then went back on and cleared her face in a week

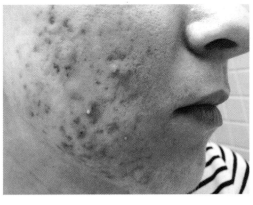

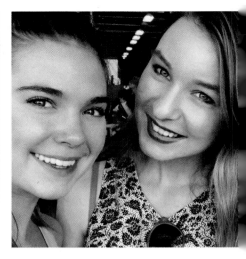

Katarina cleared her acne in 3 months

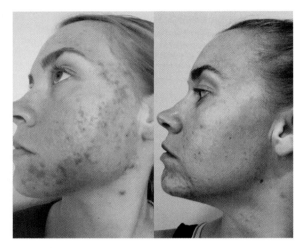

Rachel 3 months on the diet

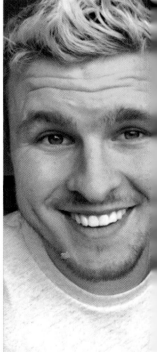

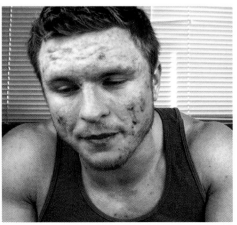

Brian Turner.
Vegetables
cleared his acne

acne-promoting effects of milk could be eliminated. At the end of the four-week period they found that dark chocolate does indeed promote acne. They documented their findings with graphic before and after photos showing the breakouts caused by chocolate. The researchers concluded: "Dark chocolate when consumed in normal amounts for four weeks can exacerbate acne in male subjects with acne-prone skin."[1]

While the Clear Skin Diet does allow fat-free cocoa powder, it doesn't allow full-fat chocolate. Below is a label for the kind of chocolate used in this study.

This label is for a 50-gram bar of 99 percent dark chocolate; study participants consumed a 25-gram bar each day, so half this amount. If you analyze this label, as we've just shown, you see that this chocolate bar has 83 percent calories from fat. That's about the same percentage of calories from fat as nuts, avocados, or other high-fat plant foods excluded on the Clear Skin Diet. The researchers who published this new study noted in the study's conclusion that it was most likely the high-fat content of the dark chocolate that caused the acne. In 1969, Dr. Fulton thought chocolate and food had nothing to do with acne. In 2016, researchers have shown that food actually does have a great deal to do with acne.

Nutrition Facts Valeur nutritive	
Per 1 bar (50 g) / pour 1 barre (50 g)	
Amount Teneur	% Daily Value % valeur quotidienne
Calories / Calories 270	
Fat / Lipides 25 g	38 %
Saturated / saturés 15 g + Trans / trans 0 g	75 %
Cholesterol / Cholestérol 0 mg	
Sodium / Sodium 20 mg	1 %
Carbohydrate / Glucides 4 g	1 %
Fibre / Fibres 3 g	12 %
Sugars / Sucres 1 g	
Protein / Protéines 7 g	
Vitamin A / Vitamine A	0 %
Vitamin C / Vitamine C	0 %
Calcium / Calcium	6 %
Iron / Fer	20 %

SODIUM

We mentioned that we recommend looking for low-salt or salt-free canned and packaged foods, when possible. Let's take a second to talk about why. Westerners consume a lot of salt, and it's not particularly good for our health. Salt makes your body retain water, and if you consume too much salt, the extra water raises your blood pressure. The higher your blood pressure, the greater the strain on your heart, arteries, kidneys, and brain. This can over time lead to heart attacks, strokes, dementia, and kidney disease. Reducing the amount of sodium you take in is a good idea.

Much of the sodium people consume comes in the form of cheese and meats—animal products. Since you'll no longer be consuming those on the

Clear Skin Diet, you're making a positive change in this department. According to the National Academy of Science, our daily requirement for sodium based on physiological need is about 250 mg per day. If we only ate fruits and vegetables and no processed food, we would get about 500 mg of sodium a day. Plant eaters are safer from sodium, while most Americans are eating between 3,000 and 5,000 mg a day. This is far too high.

Much of the high levels of sodium people consume come from restaurant food and processed foods. Eliminate or minimize those, and you will automatically be eating much less sodium.

When preparing food, we recommend that you do not ever cook with salt. Omit salt from a recipe and instead shake salt on the food just before you eat it. This will give you the biggest bang—salty taste effect—for the lowest amount of sodium. If you add salt when cooking your food, you will get a less salty taste, so you're getting more sodium for less enjoyment.

Salt is an appetite promoter. By adding salt you will be stimulated to consume more food. While we recommend many salt-free spices and mixes, lowering salt is not as critical for healing acne as lowering fat is. The Clear Skin Diet has more leeway when it comes to salt and higher sodium condiments. We want you to eat the healthy starch-based food, and if sprinkling a bit of salt or sugar helps the medicine go down, go for it.

How much sodium is too much? The upper limit set for sodium intake by the Institute of Medicine is 2,300 mg/day for healthy people age nine to fifty and 1,500 mg/day for people age fifty-one and over, as well as for African Americans and people with diabetes, hypertension, or chronic kidney disease. But as noted, 90 percent of Americans exceed the upper limit every day.

For the purposes of label reading, we recommend 1 mg of salt per calorie as an acceptable level. If you are looking at a label and it shows a serving is 100 calories, and the label lists 100 mg of sodium or less per serving, that's great. That's an ideal ratio: 1 mg of sodium per 1 calorie of food.

The allowed limit for sodium in condiments is much higher because you don't consume as much of a condiment as you do of a food, so the sodium content is not as critical. Ketchup or mustard, for example, could have a ratio of 5 mg of sodium for every one calorie of food, and that would be acceptable because they are condiments. But again, you don't have to go crazy on salt limits on the Clear Skin Diet. Just be extremely careful with fat intake; that's what's causing the acne.

CHANGING FOOD LABELS

There has been a movement recently to change the layout of the U.S. Nutrition Facts label and enhancing what information is featured on the label. Some companies have already changed their labels in anticipation of newly proposed rules. But this is a very slow process. When and if the label rules officially change, then the instructions in this book may no longer apply entirely. We will keep our website at ClearSkinDiet.com updated with any new information.

12

RESTAURANTS AND TRAVEL

by Randa

"Hey, let's go out." Whenever you hear someone say that, they are usually talking about going out to eat, not on a hike. And certainly the experience of eating in a nice restaurant, where the food is prepared for you and you can socialize with your friends and family, is one we all enjoy. Americans love to eat out. In fact, according to the US Bureau of Labor Statistics, for the first time in history, between 2015 and 2016, Americans spent more money on restaurant food than they did on groceries. But there is a price we pay for that kind of consumption—both in our pocketbooks and our health. Restaurant food typically has a 300 percent markup over homemade food. Think about 300 percent. This means something that would cost you five dollars to prepare at home would cost you fifteen dollars to eat at a restaurant. And then there is your health to consider. Restaurant food tends to have significantly more fat, sodium, and calories than home-cooked meals.

Realistically, this means that the most reliable and safest way for you to eat is to cook your own food. This is the only way you know absolutely what you're putting into your body and can be confident you're doing it right. We understand that the art of cooking has been largely lost in our culture, but it is easier than you might think to put a delicious, healthy, and satisfying meal together. Your picking up this book and learning how to apply its concepts is a huge step in the right direction—toward your kitchen. (You remember the kitchen: it's that place where you used to store your takeout!)

Batch cooking and freezing, once you master it, will make your life easier. It's faster to reheat than to drive somewhere to order and pick up or even to have something delivered. Even if you're not going to be eating at home, consider packing a lunch or dinner when you go out so you can continue to stick to the program.

ACNE ADVICE:
From Jeff Novick, MS, RD

Always plan ahead and bring food with you on any extended trip. Whether it's your car, a train, a bus, or a plane, bring enough food to cover your trip and your initial arrival period. When you arrive, find a local grocery store and get your favorite healthful foods that you can prepare simply where you are staying. If you are staying in a hotel, always look for one that has a mini kitchen with a refrigerator stove or microwave. If not, you can always use the coffee pot to make hot water to heat up the simple foods you bring or buy. If you are staying with family or friends, ask if you can have kitchen access.

Check websites like www.happycow.net to see if there are any local grocers or restaurants specializing in healthful food. Today, you can often see their menus and nutrition information at their websites. Be careful at vegan restaurants and health food stores as their food is not always healthful but can be very tempting. We often develop what has been called the health halo effect in these stores and restaurants, and we overestimate the healthfulness of the items there.

People have to go to school or work. Traveling and going out with friends are a regular part of most people's lives. Learning how to eat the Clear Skin Diet in restaurants will help you stay on track.

Here are some tips for eating out.

- ❖ Limit eating out in general (save money and your health).
- ❖ Research the online menu of a restaurant you're going to, or call ahead to ask questions.
- ❖ *Always ask questions* of your waiter or server. Make it clear their answers are important and need to be accurate. If they seem like they're not sure, ask them to please go talk to the chef and then give you an accurate answer.
- ❖ Make sure there are no animal products, no dairy, and no oil in any dish you order. Always clarify that this is extremely important to you. I remember growing up and ordering food at Disneyland

and when I would say "no dairy," sometimes the server would ask me, "Are you allergic?" I thought it was an odd question because if someone doesn't want dairy, it shouldn't matter why. But I do say I'm allergic because dairy is inflammatory, and I don't want it in my body. Don't be embarrassed to say you're allergic; that way the server is more likely to be careful and confirm with the chef that your food is clean.

- Again, one of the biggest issues when you eat out is not just animal products but oil. Many restaurants pour oil on just about everything. Be sure to investigate so you can avoid that oil. Oil can set back your progress on the anti-acne diet.
- Consider eating at home before you go out, if you're concerned there may not be good options available to you. Sometimes we eat a full meal and then just order something minor like a side dish at the actual dinner because we're already full. We're basically socially eating while other people are having their meals. This is fine, as we've already eaten 90 percent of our meal before we even arrived at the restaurant.
- Many restaurants offer salad, steamed veggies, beans, baked potatoes, rice, fruit. You can assemble a fabulous meal with those ingredients. Again, just make sure no oil, dairy, butter, or other high-fat items are used in preparation.
- Ask if they have any vegan soups: black bean soup, split pea soup, vegetable soup, minestrone, lentil soup. Again, always ask if they contain any meat, soy, or dairy products or whether they were made with oil or other fats.
- Assume many sauces, dressings, and marinades have oil, and be sure to ask the waiter before you use any. Avoid any oily sauces and ask for vinegar and lemons, limes, hot sauce, or ketchup to make a dressing.
- Ask whether bread or other appetizers contain any dairy or oil.
- Stick to your eating plan: you can always eat more when you get home, if the restaurant doesn't offer your kind of food.
- Don't be ashamed to ask questions about your food or to even be insistent about what you are eating. It's your body, remember, and you have the right and responsibility to treat it the way you want it to be treated.

Here are some specific thoughts about different kinds of restaurants and what to aim for and what to avoid:

ACNE ADVICE:
From Mary McDougall

People fail to find healthy restaurant meals when they don't commit to eat right before they look at the menu. When faced with less-than-ideal food selections, choose white rice and white bread over animal products and greasy foods. We can find a healthy, great-tasting meal for ourselves in eight out of ten restaurants. For breakfast, John orders a whole grain cold cereal with fruit juice or hot oatmeal, hash brown potatoes cooked without grease and topped with salsa or ketchup, whole wheat toast and jelly, fresh fruit, and herbal tea. For lunch and dinner, we look for a vegetarian restaurant and stay away from the eggs, cheese, and oil on their menu. Chinese, Thai, and Japanese restaurants can easily make an oil-free, animal-free topping to go over rice (usually white rice). Indian restaurants have a tradition of vegetarian cooking: tell the waiter to "hold the ghee" (clarified butter).

Chefs at most fine dining establishments consider cooking you a pure vegetarian dish with no oil to be a welcome challenge—if you give them notice. Fast meals can be had at salad bars, just leave out the selections with mayonnaise and olive oil. Many Mexican restaurants can put together a burrito or tostada made with oil-free pinto or black beans, lettuce, tomatoes, and salsa. Pizza without the cheese is almost perfect, except for the oil in the crust and the white flour. Top with generous amounts of tomato sauce and vegetables. Jusk ask. You'll be surprised how happy most restaurants are to have your business.

Mexican Restaurants

- ✧ Avoid chips (they're fried in oil) and guacamole (high fat).
- ✧ Ask for soft corn tortillas instead, if they do not contain oil (generally corn tortillas are not made with oil or fat, unlike wheat tortillas, but if corn tortillas are "hard," they may have been fried in oil in order to make them crispy, so ask).
- ✧ Consider asking for a large plain house salad with no dressing (use salsa as dressing), whole beans (not refried, which contain oil), steamed or grilled veggies, without oil, possibly brown rice, corn, or quinoa if they don't contain oil or other fatty ingredients.
- ✧ Combine the above into a colorful salad or ask for corn tortillas

and make tacos. The danger in many Mexican restaurants is oil—veggies, beans, or rice fried on an oily griddle. Request that your food is cooked on a dry griddle. Avoid cheese and sour cream, obviously.

Italian Restaurants

✧ Avoid bread (unless you're sure there's no dairy).
✧ Try the house salad with vinegar and lemon (unless they have fat-free, oil-free dressing).
✧ Minestrone or pasta fagioli soup are great options, but often they are made in chicken broth or have oil so always ask.
✧ Consider whole wheat pasta (if available) with veggies and marinara sauce.

BBQ Restaurants

✧ Consider a BBQ chicken chopped salad, minus the chicken, cheese, or ranch dressing. Usually this means greens, beans, and veggies. Top it with some vegan no-oil barbecue sauce, if available.
✧ Consider having a baked potato, side of beans, a house salad, and a side of steamed veggies. You can eat the Clear Skin Diet at steak houses like Outback Steakhouse, with some thought. Check to make sure no oil is used in anything and, of course, no butter, sour cream, or other animal products.

Chinese and Thai Restaurants

✧ Thai restaurants often will cook to order, so you are in a good position to get a decent meal. Order brown rice and steamed veggies (no oil, of course). Top with fat-free sauce.
✧ Veggie soups or curries work well, as long as they're vegan with no oil.
✧ Spring rolls or veggie rolls can be incredible if they're fresh and not deep-fried. Hot and sour soup or regular veggie soup can be a great pick, as long as the veggie broth is no oil.
✧ Order a noodle dish with clear skin ingredients only, or a veggie pad thai minus the tofu or higher fat foods and no oil. Sweet and sour veggie dishes can often be made very low fat.

Indian Restaurants

✧ There are many bean- or lentil-based veggie dishes in Indian cuisine, such as *chana masala* or dal. Ask if they are vegan or can be made vegan, and make sure they do not contain dairy or oil. Many restaurants will accommodate you and make it vegan; just be sure there is also no oil.

✧ Ask for brown rice.

ACNE ADVICE:
From Rip Esselstyn

When going out to eat or traveling, I always follow my FAB protocol:

F: Figure out what you can eat depending where you are—there's always something. Rice, steamed veggies, potatoes, sides of everything. You can do it!

A: Ask for what you want. Be specific and ask to speak to a chef or cook when you can. Then explain what you'd like to eat (and what you do not eat). I've never been to a restaurant that wasn't happy to accommodate my request.

B: Bring your own food. When you're on the road, you have to be prepared and have food with you that is compliant with your plant-strong way of eating. If you're not prepared, your willpower will be greatly diminished. Stay fueled with plant-strong goodness.

Whole Foods Markets or Supermarkets

✧ Many grocery stores have a deli area with a salad bar and/or hot food. For example, at most Whole Foods Markets, you can assemble a salad of greens and assorted vegetables, rice, and beans. Just be sure to read the store labels about each option, or ask an employee to make sure there's no oil. Top with fat-free sauces, ketchup, lemon, or vinegar.

Chain Restaurants

✧ Many chain restaurants have options that will work beautifully with the Clear Skin Diet. Panera, with over two thousand outlets in forty-six states, offers steel-cut oatmeal for breakfast, many salad options, soup options (garden vegetable or black bean), fruit, and smoothies.

✧ Wendy's offers a baked potato and steamed broccoli (hold the sour cream).

✧ Soup and salad restaurants like Souplantation feature large salad bars. Tip: make your own and avoid their premade salads, which may contain oil or animal products. Use vinegars and/or lemon juice for dressing (or lemon wedges). They sometime have vegan soups—check for oil. Some will have baked white or sweet potatoes. Top with salsa, hot sauce, lemon juice, veggies, or soup.

✧ Steak houses like Sizzler in the West have great salad bars, which usually have rice, beans, *pico de gallo*, salsa, and fruit. Use vinegars and/or lemon juice for dressing; avoid oil.

ACNE ADVICE:
From Chef AJ

One of my favorite travel tips is to buy an inexpensive cooler and to always make sure it's filled with healthy, compliant food (cooked sweet potatoes, for example, which make a delicious snack, even cold). Many of these coolers are very fashionable and even look exactly like a woman's purse so you can bring them into movie theaters without anyone taking your food!

PLANES, TRAINS, AND AUTOMOBILES

The key to traveling is this: plan ahead. Assume there's going to be nothing you can eat at the airport, on the airplane, in the gas station, and so forth. Your success depends on thinking ahead. For traveling we generally make food the night before. We think about what we're going to eat for each meal and bring it with us. That way, when we start getting hungry, we're covered. There's no challenge, no temptation to eat less-than-desirable food. We may make burritos or sandwiches, steam up a big bag of potatoes and sauce, and get bags of cherries or other fruit or 100 percent fruit bars for snacks. It's crucial you plan ahead and bring your own food. You want to feel confident going into the unknown, and the way to do that is keep yourself fed and happy. Use stainless containers or plastic bags to store your food.

---◇---

13

DORMS, DINING HALLS, AND SCHOOL

by Nina

You're away from home, you're in college—congratulations! It's the ideal time to adopt the Clear Skin Diet, heal your skin, and become the healthiest version of you possible. The first thing to know is that you're probably not alone. More and more college students are deciding to go vegan these days, for their health, for environmental concerns, or for animals. You can likely find kindred souls on campus, in your psych class, your dorm, or at the gym. There's probably a vegan group on campus, which might be worth checking out. It all depends on your interests, but nothing beats having friends with the same aims and desires. There might be other Clear Skin Diet friends-to-be on your campus, waiting to get to know you.

Here are some strategies for helping ensure you're successful at school.

EAT IN YOUR DORM ROOM OR APARTMENT

If you have a fridge in your apartment you are lucky! If you're in a dorm, consider getting a mini-fridge in your room. You can keep fresh, healthy foods on hand in order to live the clear skin way.

Then think about getting creative with a microwave and/or hot plate in your dorm. You can actually do most of your clear skin eating with just those appliances. They can be a very important investment for you.

Shop at your local discount supermarket, like Smart & Final or Costco, for good prices on fruits, veggies, and starch. Or there may be local produce markets where you can save some money while supporting local growers. Farmers' markets can often be less expensive than buying produce at supermarkets. Look for a Trader Joe's, Food 4 Less, or low-priced grocery store where you can get other staples on a budget.

Keep fruits and veggies on hand for snacks and meals. Oranges, apples, bananas, dates, carrots, celery, broccoli, spinach, potatoes, and sweet potatoes are easy go-to foods. Precooked rice you can heat up fast in your microwave anytime, which is useful in an emergency. Hungry for a satisfying, healthy meal? Take a russet or larger potato or two, poke some holes in them with a fork, put them in the microwave, and hit "potato" (or microwave at full power for five minutes). The fork holes around the potato are to keep it from rupturing as the steam tries to escape and will help it cook evenly. If you have an oven, you can even transfer the microwaved potatoes into the oven, preheated to 420 degrees F, and let the potato skins get crispy by baking them for ten to twenty minutes.

Canned beans can be a lifesaver. We always keep them on hand even when we have fresh, dried beans available to cook. Canned beans are something you can use on a hungry moment's notice, combined with rice, pasta, bread, or potato. Keep a supply of canned soups, pasta sauce, cereal, rice, quinoa, and pasta (all fat-free varieties). These foods have long shelf lives and won't go bad for a while (keep checking expiration dates and make sure you use them before they expire). Replenish them as you eat them so you'll never run out.

Oatmeal is a meal you can eat anytime of the day or night, so keep plenty of oats on hand. Put a big scoopful into a large Pyrex bowl, add water, and then hit "reheat" on your microwave. Great for breakfast, or after a late-night study session. Add some frozen berries to the steaming oatmeal, and after a few minutes they'll be melting and be a perfect topping.

Recommendations: Igloo 3.2—cu. Mini fridge; Westinghouse 900 watt counter top mini microwave; Whole Foods 365 brand canned beans

PRESSURE COOKER

Electric pressure cookers, like the Instant Pot, are around seventy dollars for a small unit. Think of it this way. It's about the same price as a textbook but could be an even better long-term investment. What do you spend to eat out and have a decent meal over the course of a year? Now compare that to investing in a pressure cooker, which will allow you to make a variety of delicious meals, all year long. If you have decided to make your skin and your health a high priority, then invest in some kitchen tools that will help you succeed. When we had severe acne and were going to the dermatologist regularly, we ended up paying hundreds of dollars for expensive prescriptions, in the hopes that they would help our complexions. The cost of a pressure cooker is minor compared to other types of skin interventions, so consider this as you decide where your priorities lie.

Recommendation: Instant Pot three-quart mini.

EAT FROZEN

School is a place where frozen fruits and veggies can rule! Once again, the microwave is your friend, and you can warm up some canned beans, potato (or rice), or your frozen veggies, and you'll have a tasty, satisfying meal. Add a little ketchup or barbecue or soy sauce. Experiment with different condiments and starches to keep these basic meals interesting and varied.

Recommendation: Bulk frozen veggies.

SNACKS

Take food with you whenever you head for class, for a workout, or for late-night studying. You never want to be stuck somewhere hungry without a meal in sight. Fruit is a great go-to snack, so carry apples, bananas, peaches, or 100 percent fruit bars. Store them in your backpack, purse, or jacket. Don't allow yourself to become ravenous because your plans suddenly changed and it's not possible to get back to your room to eat. Keep fresh water on hand in your room. If your tap water is less than appealing, consider purchasing a water filter or filtered pitcher of some sort.

Recommendation: Fresh fruit, Trader Joe's Fruit Bars; see Recipes for more snack ideas.

EXPLORE

Check out the eateries around campus. Source each one that fits with the Clear Skin Diet. Learn where you can get a snack or meal and what the hours are. Use www.happycow.net to locate vegan and veg-friendly restaurants and stores in your area. Depending on options out there for you, you may be able to work in some meals or snacks at places around you. Or you may need to be prepared to pack your lunch every day.

Recommendation: Check menus online, call ahead.

THE CAFETERIA

If you're going to attempt the cafeteria route, try to have a direct discussion with the chef and cafeteria manager. In fact, do your utmost to treat them really well and become fast friends. You want the people who control the food to become your biggest allies. Let them know you're on a special vegan diet due to your allergies (you're allergic to acne!), and figure out what they can do. Could they cook one special dish for you that's "legal"? Could they prepare plain brown rice without oil? Perfect! Perhaps bake you dry potatoes and steamed veggies on the side? Outstanding! How about beans? Plain pasta? If their sauce has oil but the pasta doesn't, you're halfway there. Just supply your own bottle of fat-free sauce. Some schools may be more accommodating than others, but it can't hurt to ask. And people definitely respond to allergies.

ACNE ADVICE:
From Jeff Novick, MS, RD

Focus on yourself. Until you understand the program, put the time in over the next few months, and achieve and maintain your own success, keep the focus and attention on yourself. Don't be swayed by the opinions of others, the news of the day, or trying to explain your dietary choices or get others to do it. Keep the focus on understanding and implementing the program and getting your skin healed. Don't become an evangelist or try to convert anyone. Taking care of yourself is not selfish; this is self-nurturing, and right now, you need all your focus and attention on you.

Avoid the vegan trap. Vegan is now a popular trend, but this is not always good news. While this is good for the animals and the environment, most of the vegan food in grocery stores and restaurants is not healthful. The Pleasure Trap appeal of many of these unhealthful vegan foods is strong and can be hard to resist.

DORM KITCHEN

Some dorms have a kitchen for public use, usually used for a party or event. Take advantage of the space and use it for batch cooking. When you have some extra time, cook a variety of starches or roast a bunch of veggies, and then store them in glass or plastic containers in your fridge or freezer. This could set you up completely for the upcoming week.

Recommendation: Explore using the dorm kitchen.

REPETITION EQUALS SUCCESS

Discover the foods you prefer, and then find a way to make those meals repeatedly. Spend an afternoon experimenting with the recipes in this book, and try to find your favorites. Then you can add that into your rotation of the four, six, or eight meals that comprise your diet. There's no need to have a great variety. It's about what works, what satisfies, and what you can prepare easily.

Recommendation: Wash, rinse, repeat

EDUCATE YOURSELF

You've made a big leap, both by reading this book and then embracing a healthy plant-based diet. When you are ready, try reading some books by additional plant-based experts. There are several interesting documentaries about the health benefits of plant-based eating, which you may enjoy. (See Resources section for suggestions.) The more educated you become about the clear skin lifestyle, the more motivated you'll become, helping assure your success.

Recommendation: You're in school already, so read some more!

14

WEIGHT MAINTENANCE

by Randa

If you have been eating like most Americans, expect some positive changes to your health after you start following the Clear Skin Diet. Acne will calm, slow, and then halt. Your skin will finally begin to heal. An additional side effect could be weight loss. Why? Because the foods you're going to be emphasizing—healthy fruits, vegetables, whole grains, and legumes—are lower-calorie foods than you may be accustomed to.

One way to categorize foods is by how many calories they contain per pound. Some foods have very few calories, like vegetables (an average of 100 calories per pound). Some foods contain a lot of calories, like nuts (2,800 calories per pound). Processed oils, like olive or canola oil, are the most calorie-loaded foods in existence (4,000 calories per pound).

Most weight loss diets work through portion control. To lose weight, you need to create a calorie deficit, and by eating smaller portions, you are cutting the amount of calories you're taking in. That makes you lose weight. For example, let's say you restrict portions so that you eat 500 fewer calories per day than your body burns. In the space of a week you would be short 3,500 calories (seven days times 500 calories less per day). A pound equals 3,500 calories, so theoretically you're going to lose a pound a week if you're taking in 500 fewer calories per day than you're burning.

On the Clear Skin Diet, you are going to forget about counting calories. Calorie counting seems to make people crazy and obsessive about their food. We want you to feel happy and confident that each bite you put in your mouth is wholesome and good—because it is. And when you emphasize the foods we recommend, you'll be eating a diet that is already naturally very low in calories. Unprocessed plant foods are among the lowest in calorie density. By filling up on these low-calorie foods, you're going to be "crowding out" higher-calorie foods. These whole plant foods also help keep your blood sugar balanced and keep hunger pangs at bay. With the Clear Skin Diet, you can eat until you're full and still lose weight, and you can stop worrying.

Here is a chart that shows calories per pound of recommended foods from the Clear Skin Diet:

CALORIES PER POUND	CALORIE DENSITY
100 CALS.	VEGETABLES (NON-STARCHY)
300 CALS.	FRUIT
400 CALS.	POTATO, CORN, SQUASH, OATS
500 CALS.	WHOLE GRAINS, RICE, PASTA
600 CALS.	BEANS & LEGUMES
750 CALS.	AVOCADOS
1000 CALS.	MEATS
1200 CALS.	ICE CREAM
1400 CALS.	BREAD/BAGELS/WRAPS
1600 CALS.	CHEESE, DRY CEREAL
1800 CALS.	SUGAR, CRACKER POPCORN
2500 CALS.	CHOCOLATE
2800 CALS.	NUTS, SEEDS, BUTTERS, TAHINI
4000 CALS.	ALL OILS, OILPOPPED POPCORN

The first five food groups are the primary foods you will eat on the Clear Skin Diet. They range in calorie density from 100 calories per pound (non-starchy vegetables) to 600 calories per pound (beans and legumes). Most people eating the standard American or standard Western diets are going to be attracted to higher-calorie foods, regularly eating things like meat and chicken (1,000 calories/pound), ice cream (1,200 calories/pound), cheese (1,600 calories per pound), chocolate (2,500 calories per pound). A lot of their meals might be prepared with oil (4,000 calories per pound). What inevitably happens is that they end up eating significantly more calories than people following the Clear Skin Diet, even when they eat the exact same volume of food.

The concept of eating by calorie density is also sometimes called volumentrics. By focusing on foods lower in calories and getting full and satisfied on those foods, we kick out richer foods higher in calories. In other words, we eat a lot of food but don't take in excess calories.

ACNE ADVICE:
From Matthew Lederman, MD

Remember that taste buds can evolve so you can easily get used to lower-calorie foods, just as long as you don't stimulate your taste buds again with high-calorie foods. People on a calorie-dense diet are effectively overstimulating their pleasure receptors (designed to seek out calorie density in an effort to get you the most calories with the least amount of effort). When switching to a healthier, lower-calorie (normal) diet, you may go through a period of withdrawal.

After years of overstimulation on the standard American diet (where foods with a calorie density of 2,000, 3,000, and even 4,000 calories per pound are consumed), your taste buds initially crave those calorie-dense foods and associated pleasure stimulation. However, if you stay the course and trust that these healthier, lower-calorie foods are the exact foods your body has evolved to consume over millions of years, then over time your taste buds will change and be able to achieve similar pleasure from the less stimulating, lower-calorie foods. The key here is that you must trust that this will happen and not expose your taste buds and pleasure receptors to the older hyperstimulating foods. Just as an ex-drug addict cannot "taste" heroin again, you should not taste overstimulating, high-calorie, dense, processed junk foods. If you do, you will reverse the neuro-adaptation or "evolution" that has already happened and then have to reacclimate your taste buds to the healthier, lower-calorie foods once again. This not only takes time but also is unpleasant—so why torture yourself?

The clear skin versions of sauces, condiments, bread, and desserts are higher in calorie density than our staple food, but that is OK. You can also have bagels, popcorn, cereals, and pancakes, which are also higher-calorie foods. The foundation of the Clear Skin Diet are those foods that are 600 calories per pound or less, such as starches, fruits, vegetables, whole grains, rice, pasta, beans, and all the foods that are health promoting, though. When you start consuming these calorie-light foods, your body will naturally start adjusting to its ideal weight, without your really thinking about it. Forget about the scale; remember your veggies.

If you're a survivor of the standard meat-heavy, dairy-laden, oily diet, there will be an adjustment to eating a new way. If for some reason this doesn't work for you—perhaps you are already very slim and don't want to lose any weight—use the Calorie Density Chart in reverse to add in more calorie-dense plant foods. To gain weight or prevent weight loss, eat more foods that are higher in calorie density, like dried fruits (much higher calorie density because the water's been removed), bread, and other processed grains like dry cereals, crackers, and pasta (processing food makes it more calorie dense). Add high-calorie foods like maple syrup to your oatmeal and pancakes, and add liquid calories like juices and smoothies with dates (which will increase caloric intake).

Another way to look at this concept of calorie density is to consider the amount of food your stomach can hold. Your brain tells you to stop eating when you hit a certain level of satiety and a certain level of physical fullness. Look at the following graphic, which shows how much 500 calories of each of these foods would look like in your stomach.

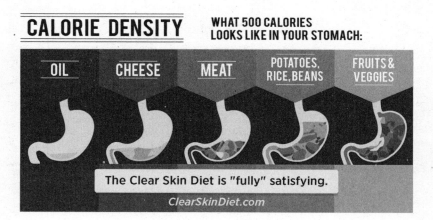

To take in 500 calories into your stomach, you could have 2 ounces of olive oil, or 4 ounces of cheese, or 8 ounces of meat, or 17 ounces of rice, beans and potatoes, or 53 ounces of veggies. The average stomach holds between 35 and 50 ounces, so you can see you can get very full on potatoes, rice, beans, and veggies, but it's going to take a *lot* more calories of oil, cheese, and meat to get that same feeling of fullness.

In general you don't have to think about your weight when you start eating the clear skin way. Over time your body will find the ideal weight it wants to be. But again, if you're trying to lose weight, use calorie density as your guide, and you won't have to count or limit how much you're eating. You're already eating lower calories when you follow the Clear Skin Diet.

Most importantly, don't think about weight or weight loss starting out. Just focus on following the diet and being satisfied. We like to tell people to think "health gain" and not "weight loss."

It is important, though, to realize that starches are naturally low in calories and high in satiation, meaning they make you feel full and satisfied. This is the reason you can always eat the clear skin way. Think of a big plate of mashed potatoes with gravy and maybe some corn or peas on top. We call it comfort food because it's very satisfying. In fact, in studies potatoes rank number one on the satiety index, meaning they are the most satiating food we eat.[1]

There's a lot of research on potatoes going back more than a hundred years, showing they are an ideal food nutritionally. In 1913 a Danish physician and pioneering nutritionist named Mikkel Hindhede proved you could survive on potatoes alone—in fact you could *thrive* on a potato-only diet.

Dr. McDougall often talks about a study done in 1925 where researchers took two healthy people, a twenty-five-year-old man and a twenty-eight-year-old woman, and put them on a diet for six months of primarily white potatoes. They were also allowed to have butter on their potatoes for extra calories, some coffee and tea, and occasional fruits. But the bulk of the diet was potatoes. Researchers reported that at the end of six months, the man and woman had never tired of their diet; they never craved other foods. They were tested for protein levels and health biomarkers and were determined to be in excellent health on a potato-only diet. They were also able to do as much intense physical activity as they wished.

WHY DO STARCHES ENCOURAGE WEIGHT LOSS?

Generally speaking, a gram of fat has nine calories, while a gram of carbohydrate and protein each have four calories. As a carbohydrate, a gram of white sugar contains four calories, but a gram of potato, which includes a lot of fiber, has only about one calorie. That means you can eat a lot of potatoes—mashed, baked, roasted, or boiled—and not be consuming many calories.

The same is true of many carbohydrates, even some breads, cereals, and other more calorie-dense foods. You can still lose weight with these foods. People are skeptical when they hear bread might be a weight-loss food, and Dr. McDougall often cites a study of bread done by researchers from the Food Science and Human Nutrition Department at Michigan State University. Researchers took sixteen overweight college-age men and told them to add twelve slices of white bread (seventy calories a slice) or twelve slices of high-fiber bread (fifty calories a slice) to their diet every day. Over the next eight weeks, the men eating the extra white bread lost an average of fourteen pounds while those who added the high-fiber bread to their regular diet lost nineteen pounds. There was no change in the men's exercise or other physical activity level. Their weight loss was purely as a result of diet.[2]

Not only did the men lose weight, their cholesterol went down—just from adding the extra bread to their diet. The moral of the story? Don't fear carbs! Men in the Michigan State study added twelve slices of bread, or 840 extra calories from bread per day, and lost weight! They weren't adding jam or jelly or any high-calorie spreads on their bread; they just ate the extra bread. The fullness they got from that bread seems to have crowded out other higher-calorie foods they might have eaten instead. The bread wasn't the problem for these overweight college men. They lost pounds because the bread displaced the fat-heavy burgers, fries, cheese pizza, and other animal products.

Starches—like rice, corn, potatoes, beans, oatmeal, pasta, and even bread—can help return you to an optimal weight, without counting calories. Isn't it a relief to learn that comfort foods like these are actually our natural, healthiest diet? Again, it's when you add the fatty foods—the oils, the eggs, the ice cream, the sausages, the fried chicken—that weight becomes a problem, your general health suffers, and your complexion starts having issues.

SCIENTIFIC PROOF CLEAR SKIN DIET PROMOTES WEIGHT LOSS

The specific diet style you're embarking on has been rigorously studied for healthy and realistic weight loss goals. The Royal New Zealand College of General Practice enrolled thirty-three participants who had been diagnosed with obesity or overweight. The participants had also been diagnosed with at least one of the following: type 2 diabetes, ischaemic heart disease, hypertension, or hypercholesterolaemia. Researchers put them on a Clear Skin–style diet for twelve weeks and told participants not to count calories and not to increase their exercise during the study period. Six months after doing the twelve-week program, participants had lost an average of 12.1 kilograms (or over 26 pounds) and reversed their medical conditions. One year after the program had ended, participants had maintained a loss of 11.5 kilograms (about 25 pounds). Participants also reported they felt they had higher self-esteem and nutritional know-how, and had lower cholesterol.[3] Learning to eat by Clear Skin Diet principles can help you achieve optimal weight and health.

ACNE ADVICE:
From John McDougall, MD

Fats taken in excess of daily needs are handled adeptly by the body. Since they are already in the chemical form for storage, they are simply moved from the fork and spoon to the fat cells. The process is so efficient that the fats retain their original chemical structure. A needle biopsy of your fatty tissue would reveal the kinds of foods you like. If you eat lots of cold-water marine fish, then your fatty tissues will be full of omega-3 fats. If you like margarine, you will be full of trans fats.

FEEL LIKE BINGEING?

A participant in one of our Acne Intervention Programs, Jazmin, disclosed that after a couple weeks into the program, she was consumed by an overwhelming desire to have a burger and milkshake. Jazmin was thinking about going to a popular vegan restaurant here in Los Angeles where she could get a yummy (but oily) vegan burger and a delicious (but full of high-fat almond milk) vegan shake. Jazmin announced this on the private Facebook Clear Skin Diet group. Randa responded, suggesting Jazmin's desire to binge on high-calorie food might actually be a signal that Jazmin was simply not eating enough calories. Since Jazmin was not used to eating mainly low calorie-dense foods, maybe she was undereating.

Her brain was drawing her attention to high-calorie foods, making Jazmin feel like she wanted to hop in her car and go pig out. Randa suggested Jazmin go eat a second dinner at home; have some mashed potatoes with gravy, some pancakes with maple syrup, some cereal with oat milk—but not go for the high-fat vegan meal. At our next meeting Jazmin reported that Randa had been right.

ACNE ADVICE:
From Chef AJ

The best advice I can offer for staying compliant on this diet is to make sure you are eating enough food and particularly enough STARCH! You also have to give yourself some time to adjust to a lower-fat diet and for your new way of eating to become your *preferred* way of eating. This could take a month, or more, but when you see the changes in your skin and how great you feel you will be very motivated to stick with it.

She had just had more dinner and suddenly felt satisfied, no longer had any craving for junk food.

The Clear Skin Diet food is bulkier, has more fiber and more volume, and can make you feel full on fewer calories. If you start feeling hungry, eat more healthy food! Don't go on an acne-promoting food spree. Eat more healthy starches, and that will help with cravings and make you feel more balanced.

15

EXERCISE IS SELF-CARE

by Nina

Exercise helps combat acne by boosting your happiness levels, helping you set and achieve goals, and reducing your risk of serious illnesses. You sleep better, feel more energetic, and increase your strength and flexibility. Additional benefits include improving your memory, your self-confidence, and your ability to work at school or at a job. Generally, it can help extend your life and be healthy while you're living it. Exercise is an important part of the clear skin lifestyle—as it should be an important part of everyone's life.

If you already have a regular exercise routine you love, that's great! The key to any successful program is to do something you really enjoy because then you'll look forward to it and actually *do* it. I've seen people who decide they need to quickly get in shape, so they find a boot camp and get up early to line up with a group of strangers. They huff and puff and struggle and get their body pounded; they might even get injured from doing too much too fast. They end up dreading the workout because it's too early or too challenging or they get too sore—it's a chore. Attention: that is *not* what the clear skin workout is about. At all. We are about having fun and enjoying yourself, while raising your heart rate and putting some resistance against your muscles and bones.

CLEAR SKIN WORKOUT ROUTINE

We recommend you try to exercise four or five days a week, for thirty minutes to an hour. You will do cardio three times a week and some form of resistance or strength training on the other two days.

We're going to present a menu of activities that you can choose from. Pick the ones you think you'll enjoy. The key is to get a routine going, if you don't already have one. But we're not insisting that you do any particular exercises other than those you prefer. Exercise will maximize the benefits of the Clear Skin Diet program.

We encourage you to do a variety of different types of exercise over a given month. We're big believers in the concept of "muscle confusion." Muscle confusion means you don't work the same group of muscles every time you exercise. Mix it up, so that you are constantly challenging your body in new ways. One day you may swim, bike, walk, run, or jump rope; another you might try lunges and squats or resistance training. Or pick one day for high-intensity interval training. Varying your exercise routine gives your body a chance to recover from whatever you did the day before, and you also won't hit a plateau.

Some of you may have been exercising all your lives; others may be a little out of shape or haven't really been doing much regular exercise for a while. Exercises can be done at varying levels, and you should consider where you are in terms of beginner to expert athlete.

Here is a schedule of workout suggestions—which is not to say you should specifically follow this calendar. This schedule is simply an example of how your month might look, in terms of different types of activities to mix and match. Do the physical activities available to you and that you find enjoyable. Please be sure to consult your doctor before beginning any exercise program.

Sample Clear Skin Workout Routine

	Week 1	Week 2	Week 3	Week 4
Day One		Jump Rope	Weights	
Day Two	Walk	HIIT		HIIT
Day Three	Run		Run	Walk
Day Four		Swim	Walk	Run
Day Five	Weights			
Day Six	Cardio	Hike	Cardio	Bike
Day Seven	HIIT	Cardio Class	HIIT	Jump Rope

CARDIO EXERCISES

On cardio days, pick something that will get your heart rate elevated for twenty to forty minutes. Here are some possibilities:

WALKING

Walking is absolutely essential to life. When you walk you're moving oxygen around your body, increasing circulation, and elevating your heart rate. Studies have shown that moderate-intensity walking is just as effective as running for lowering risk of several chronic diseases like high blood pressure, type 2 diabetes, certain cancers, and other conditions.

RUNNING

Randa and I generally do long runs once or twice a week. Running can improve your general health, prevent diseases, stabilize weight, boost your confidence, relieve stress, and eliminate depression. It's almost magic—but only if running is something you like to do. If running is not for you, move on.

If you haven't run much recently, be sure to start out slowly, taking shorter runs to begin with. Don't run every day; give your body time to recuperate and adjust to the new activity.

BIKING

We love to bike! Be careful if you're riding on busy streets; bike trails are preferred. Biking gives your lower body muscles a great workout and is gentler on your joints than running. If you have hills around to climb, you can get an even better workout. If you use a stationary exercise bike, work harder to raise your heart rate.

SWIMMING

Swimming is a great cardio workout if you make a consistent effort to put in the laps. Swimming is low impact, is good for increasing your lung capacity, improves sleep, and increases strength.

ROWING

Most gyms have a rowing machine, and rowing can be a big cardio workout. Rowing targets large groups of muscles on both the upper and lower body. It's also low impact, which lowers the chance for injuries. Twenty or thirty minutes of intense rowing is actually quite a workout.

JUMPING ROPE

Jumping rope can be done just about anywhere, and it's so much fun. Do three or four rounds of ten minutes each. This is comparable to running at a very fast pace. It can also help on improving your balance. Start out slow and work your way up to thirty minutes.

HIGH-INTENSITY INTERVAL TRAINING

We love high-intensity interval training (HIIT). You can do HIIT anywhere, anytime, because no equipment is required—or minimal equipment for some exercises.

We use a Tabata App when we do HIIT; Tabata training consists of eight rounds of ultra-high-intensity exercises in a 20-seconds-on, 10-seconds-off interval. The Tabata App (and there are dozens of free apps) does the timing for you. Set the app for one round, and it counts down to start out. It plays for 20 seconds, during which you do the exercise with high intensity, then it counts off 10 seconds, during which you rest, and then back to 20 on, 10 off, cycling through the eight rounds.

Use the Tabata timer to turn other aerobic exercises into a HIIT exercise. For example, during the first set, you could alternate between jump squats and high knees for 20 seconds, then rest for 10 seconds, resume for 20 seconds, rest for 10, and so on, and the Tabata App tells you when to rest. For a second round, you could do jumping jacks for 20 seconds, then 10 seconds rest, push-ups for 20 seconds, then 10 seconds rest, alternating back and forth between the jumping jacks and push-ups for the eight rounds.

Tabata moves that work with the Tabata App include Mountain Climbers, Plank, Frog Jumps, Running in Place, Lunges, Fast Feet, Burpee, Side Skater, Bicycle Crunch, and Sprints.

RESISTANCE TRAINING

If you have access to a gym, you can lift weight; you can do resistance training with resistance bands. Weight lifting and resistance training both increase strength and muscle size and help tone your body. Resistance and weight training will help you burn fat more effectively. If you're doing resistance- and weight-training exercises, remember to warm up first for five to ten minutes with some cardio (like walking in place, jogging on a treadmill, or using an elliptical).

FITNESS CLASSES

If you have a gym or belong to a fitness center, there are often a variety of classes available, like Zumba, stretching, yoga, kickboxing, Pilates, toning, spin classes, dancing, which are all really fun workouts. Pick a day or two a week to have a fun aerobic workout at a gym.

DEVELOP THE HABIT OF WORKING OUT

Work to create a routine of exercising four or five days a week. Find a time of day that you can dependably get a workout: early in the morning, before lunch, in the afternoon or evening—whenever you can commit to do it. Develop the habit of sweating, raising your heart rate, and making your body feel strong by making physical demands on it. And remember: keep it fun!

PART IV

RECIPES

The six pillars of the Clear Skin Diet:

1. Plant foods only, no animal products

2. Unrefined starches should be cornerstone of your diet

3. Avoid all oils

4. Avoid high-fat plant foods

5. Eat whole foods, food as grown, minimally processed

6. Eat simply; variety is not important, repetition can promote long-term success

16

THE CLEAR SKIN RECIPES

Do you feel a bit like Dorothy knocking on the gates of Oz, ready to ask the wizard to banish your acne? Fortunately, the Clear Skin Diet does not require the use of enchantment. We are sure, however, that you will believe the food you are eating has magical powers, once you see your skin start to heal.

In this section we have categorized the recipes as follows:

Breakfasts
Handhelds: Wraps, Burritos, and Sandwiches
Soups
Bowls
Main Dishes, Entreés, Casseroles
Sauces and Gravies
Snacks and Desserts
Bonus Recipes (for plant milks and gluten-free flour mix)

But before you dive into the recipes, a word about how we have organized various types of food: please don't take these categories too literally. For instance, oatmeal is listed as a breakfast item. But hey, you can eat oatmeal whenever you crave it. The same goes for any other breakfast, like breakfast potatoes or pancakes. For that matter, you can have soup for breakfast, lentil loaf for lunch, or French toast for dinner. In other words, if you find a meal you like, it doesn't matter what time of day you eat it. Just eat that food. We had rice and beans for breakfast and cereal for dinner plenty of times growing up. Our brother used to demand split pea soup for breakfast. Nothing wrong with that! Don't be a slave to time-of-day food labels. Mix up your meals however you'd like. If you enjoy the Mushroom Bun Me recipe on page 195, take the pickled mixture and use it in a burrito, a bowl, or just as a snack. As long as you're following the Clear Skin Diet guidelines, you can be flexible with your food.

Some of the following recipes have the word *KISS* in the title: KISS is sometimes an acronym for "Keep it simple stupid." But in our book, KISS means "Keep it super simple." KISS Oatmeal, for instance, is a quick and easy way to make oatmeal. Once you learn how to make plain old oatmeal, or rice, or beans, there are endless possibilities for the recipes you can create with these items in your kitchen. On the other hand, you might be content with just plain rice, beans, and veggies. That is, in fact, pretty much our go-to meal for lunch and dinner—and sometimes breakfast! Or get a little fancy and top the rice, beans, and veggies with the Mushroom Bun Me mix. Just never be afraid to keep it super simple. It's not about making your lunch Instagram perfect. Take fifteen minutes to make lunch, and then forty-five minutes for a run—not vice versa!

And don't worry about portion control. Eat until you are satisfied. Enjoy every complexion-affirming bite.

BREAKFASTS

Is breakfast the most important meal of the day? Personally, we think every meal you eat is important. That said, according to a study published in 2005 by Tufts University, children who ate breakfast performed better academically in school. Their memory was sharper, and they were more creative. And their cognitive functions were negatively impacted when they skipped breakfast. This study also showed the type of food children ate for breakfast mattered. Those who ate a high-fiber, high-carbohydrate diet (like oatmeal and fruit) had more mental and physical energy than those who ate a higher-fat breakfast (like eggs and bacon).

So eating a good breakfast can be helpful, and our advice is to use quick and easy type recipes during the week (like oatmeal or whole grain cereal) and to get fancier and more complicated on the weekend (like waffles and pancakes).

Recommendation: Eat breakfast!

- -

KISS Cereal

1 cup whole grain cereal
½ cup homemade plant milk
Fruit of your choice

This isn't so much a recipe as more a reminder that anyone can pour cereal from a box into a bowl, splash some plant milk on it, and add some cut-up fruit. No excuse not to fix yourself breakfast! Many people are quite content with just cereal and fruit for their morning meal; just make sure it's not a cereal chock-full of sugar and unintelligible ingredients. Dry cereal with dried fruit is also a great snack, in a pinch. Throw some cereal and fruit in a baggy, and off you go.

Dry cereals should be whole grains and contain no added oils. Recommendation: Grape-Nuts, Shredded Wheat, Raisin Bran, Kamut Puffs, puffed corn, wheat, rice, and millet, various multigrain flake cereals,

- -

KISS Oatmeal

A plain old bowl of oatmeal is the absolute perfect way to start your day—or afternoon, evening, or whenever. It's a meal or a snack—filling, healthy, and easy to make.

Prep time: 5 minutes; Cook time: 3 minutes
Servings: 1 to 2

1 cup old-fashioned rolled oats
Cut fruit of choice

Combine oats and 2 cups water and heat in a microwavable glass bowl for 2 to 3 minutes. Top with fruit.
Option: Top with cinnamon, date sugar, or maple syrup. That's it!

- -

Wake Me Up before I Go Go Overnight Oats

Are you super pressed for time when you wake up? Try making your breakfast at night! We adore just about anything in a mason jar, and we love oatmeal, so we're combining the two for this no-brainer get-me-out-the-door skin-healthy meal. This a basic overnight oats recipe, followed by twelve variations, because mason jars come twelve to a case.

Prep time: 5 minutes
Servings: 1 jar equals 1 serving

16-ounce mason jar with lid
½ cup old-fashioned rolled oats
1 tablespoon Grape-Nuts
½ teaspoon vanilla
1 tablespoon maple syrup
⅛ cup raisins or other dried fruit

Mix ingredients in medium-size bowl along with 2/3 cup water or plant milk; spoon into a jar. Make sure lid is closed tightly, and refrigerate overnight.

Option: Add 2 tablespoons fat-free cocoa powder (e.g., Wonderslim): tastes like chocolate pudding.

Add ¼ cup fresh or frozen blueberries: tastes like a blueberry muffin.

Add ⅛ cup mashed sweet potato and 1 teaspoon cinnamon: tastes like sweet potato pie.

Add ⅛ cup mashed pumpkin and pumpkin pie spice: tastes like Thanksgiving!

Add juice of one lemon: tastes like lemon parfait.

Add juice of two fresh key limes and 1 tablespoon coconut sugar: tastes like key lime pie.

Add one grated carrot, and 1 teaspoon cinnamon: tastes like carrot cake.

Add ½ cup puréed frozen raspberries: tastes like breakfast sorbet.

Add ¼ cup diced apples, ¼ cup applesauce, 1 tablespoon lemon juice, and 1 teaspoon cinnamon: tastes like apple pie.

Add ½ teaspoon cinnamon and ginger powder and a pinch of ground cloves: tastes like a gingerbread cookie.

Add 1 tablespoon curry, ½ cup canned chickpeas, and ¼ cup shredded fresh spinach. This makes the oats taste more savory than sweet, but it's delicious: tastes like a touch of India.

Add 1 teaspoon turmeric, ¼ cup cooked lentils, ¼ cup shredded raw zucchini, and some fresh kale leaves: tastes like you are really making an effort to eat a super-healthy breakfast.

Overnight oats are all meant to be single serving breakfasts. If you want to make extra so you have some for a couple of days in advance, double or triple the batch. They're good for about 2 to 3 days refrigerated. You can add different variations for each day and know that you have some wonderful breakfasts to look forward to. Grab and go go!

Nina's Note: Top with a crunchy toasted oats topping. Preheat oven to 350. Spread old fashioned oats over a cookie sheet, and bake for about 10 minutes or until the oats are slightly browned and crisped. Store oats in air-tight container. This also makes a fun topping for fruit bowls, smoothies, banana ice creams, and more.

Nina's Note: We are not recommending adding bananas to the overnight mixes, as they have a tendency to turn brown, and that's just not appetizing. If you want to add fresh bananas, do it the morning of. These are all meant to be served cold.

- -

Bountiful Breakfast Rice

We want you to be inspired to sample some savory oatmeal recipes, as that may be something new and unique to your palate. We would also like to encourage you to get a little adventurous with rice—sweet rice. If it's cold outside, serve it hot; it it's warm, cool it down. It's great either way.

Prep time: 5 minutes; Cook time: 2 to 3 minutes
Servings: 1

1 cup precooked or leftover rice
⅔ cup homemade plant milk
1 small apple, chopped
¼ cup raisins
1 tablespoon maple syrup
1 teaspoon ground cinnamon/apple pie spice
2 teaspoons lemon juice

Combine all ingredients into a microwave-safe glass bowl. Stir. Cook in microwave for 2 to 3 minutes.

WEEKEND KITCHEN WARRIORS BREAKFASTS

Wanna go out for pancakes? Just don't. Please. Restaurant pancake batter is made with eggs and dairy, and then fried in oil and topped with butter. They're cute little round fat bombs. Who has time to make pancakes, anyway? You do, because the only time you're going to cook dishes like pancakes, waffles, and other more complicated breakfast recipes is when you have a day off work or school. Our advice is to stick to oatmeal and cereal Monday through Friday, and play with pancakes on the weekend.

- -

Basic Fluffy Pancakes

It's 2 a.m., and you have the day off tomorrow. That sounds to me like the perfect time for pancakes. Be sure to use a nonstick griddle pan, and don't be tempted to flip too soon.

Prep time: 15 minutes; Cook time: 15 minutes
Servings: About 6 pancakes

1 cup all-purpose flour or gluten-free flour mix, sifted
2 teaspoon baking powder
2 tablespoons maple sugar
¾ cup homemade plant milk or two mashed bananas

¼ cup chickpea flour beaten with ¼ cup water

2 tablespoons applesauce

1 tablespoon apple cider vinegar

1 teaspoon vanilla extract

In a separate bowl, mix the plant milk or bananas, chickpea flour blend, applesauce, vinegar, and vanilla.

Pour the wet ingredient mixture into the dry ingredients and mix but do not over stir. Pancake batter should be thick and slightly lumpy and not too liquidy. If it's too thick, thin it a bit with a small amount of the plant milk. Overmixing the batter can lead to hockey pucks instead of pancakes, so don't beat up the batter. Allow the batter to set for 5 to 10 minutes.

Heat a nonstick griddle (preferred method) or nonstick frying at medium high. When a few drops of water sizzle on the pan, it's time to cook. Scoop out the batter 1/4 cup at a time, and add to pan. Flip pancake when large bubbles appear through the cake. Serve with real maple syrup and fruit of your choice.

- -

Oh My Sweet Potato Pancakes

You'll find out why we call these pancakes "oh my" when you try them! It's hard to believe that something this tasty could actually be clear skin promoting, but these pancakes are full of vitamin A goodness.

Prep time: 15 minutes; Cook time: 15 minutes
Servings: About 8 pancakes

2 cups all-purpose flour or gluten-free flour mix

2 teaspoons baking powder

1 teaspoon ground cinnamon

1 teaspoon ground ginger (optional)

1½ cups homemade plant milk or 2 mashed bananas and
  applesauce

1 cup sweet potato purée

½ cup chickpea flour beaten with ½ cup flour

1 tablespoon maple syrup

2 tablespoons applesauce

1 teaspoon vanilla extract

In one bowl, mix the flour, baking powder, cinnamon, and ginger. In a separate bowl, mix the plant milk or bananas with applesauce, sweet potato purée, chickpea flour blend, maple syrup, applesauce, and vanilla extract.

Pour the wet ingredient mixture into the dry ingredients and mix. Do not overstir.

Heat a nonstick griddle or nonstick frying at medium high. Scoop out batter 1/4 cup at a time, and add to pan. Flip the pancake when large bubbles appear through the cake. Serve with real maple syrup.

Option: Use pumpkin mash instead of sweet potato.

Willie's Waffles

These waffles are named in honor of our brother, Willie, who would have eaten waffles for every meal growing up if our mom had let him. This is a Willie-approved recipe, and we hope you like it too.

Prep time: 15 minutes; Cook time: 10 minutes
Servings: About 6 waffles

1¼ cups all-purpose flour or gluten-free flour mix

2 teaspoons baking powder

½ teaspoon baking soda

1⅓ cups homemade plant milk

⅛ cup chickpea flour beaten with ⅛ cup water

1 tablespoon apple cider vinegar

2 tablespoons applesauce

1 tablespoon maple syrup

1 teaspoon vanilla extract

In one bowl mix the flour, baking powder, and baking soda. In a separate bowl, mix the plant milk, chickpea flour blend, apple cider vinegar, applesauce, maple syrup, and vanilla extract.

Pour the wet ingredient mixture into the dry ingredients and mix lightly. Let stand for about five minutes before using.

Heat a nonstick waffle maker according to the manufacturer's instructions. Pour the batter onto the waffle iron. Cooking time will depend on the waffle maker, but you want to cook your waffles until they are crispy golden-brown. Usually, when the waffle iron stops steaming, the waffles are ready.

Oh So Sweet Potato Waffles

You didn't think we'd give you a sweet potato pancake recipe and not give you a sweet potato waffle recipe as well, did you? Personally, we prefer sweet potato waffles because we love getting that extra dose of vitamin A in when we can—and they are just so dang good.

Prep time: 15 minutes; Cook time: 15 minutes
Servings: About 8 waffles

1¼ cup mashed sweet potato
1¼ cup all-purpose flour or gluten-free flour mix
¼ cup cornstarch
2 teaspoons baking powder
½ teaspoon sea salt
1 teaspoon cinnamon
1½ cups homemade plant milk or 1½ mashed
  bananas and applesauce
⅛ cup chickpea flour beaten with ⅛ cup water
1 tablespoon rice wine vinegar
⅓ cup applesauce
2 tablespoons maple syrup
1 teaspoon vanilla extract

In one bowl, mix the potato, flour, cornstarch, baking powder, sea salt, and cinnamon. In a separate bowl, mix the plant milk or bananas with applesauce, chickpea flour blend, vinegar, applesauce, maple syrup, and vanilla.

Pour the wet ingredients into the dry ingredients and mix lightly. Let stand for about 5 minutes before using.

Heat a nonstick waffle maker according to the manufacturer's instructions. Pour the batter onto the waffle iron. Cook waffles until they are crispy golden-brown. Usually, when the waffle iron stops steaming, the waffles are ready.

- -

Heavenly Hash Browns

Who doesn't love hash browns? Crispy on the outside, pillowy soft on the inside. Devour them hot off the grill, topped with ketchup, and you'll be one happy camper. Hash browns aren't quite as easy to produce as you might think, however. If you just peel your potatoes and shred them with a cheese grater, you will end up with a gray gooey mess before they even hit the griddle. Not to worry, we have cracked the hash-brown code. With just a few extra easy steps, you can produce the hash browns you dream of (and we know you do) in a few minutes.

Prep time: 10 minutes; Cook time: 15 to 20 minutes
Servings: About 4

3 large russet potatoes, peeled
Ice water
Salt and pepper

The reason your raw, shredded potatoes turn all gray and gross is because they have oxidized. There is a way around this, though. Set aside a large mixing bowl filled with ice water. As you peel each potato, set it in the bowl. The ice water will halt the oxidization while you finish peeling. Once your potatoes are all peeled, shred them one at a time in a food processor, not a cheese shredder. The quicker you shred the potatoes, the less time they have to become oxidized. Don't even bother with the cheese shredder, seriously; it takes forever, and the potatoes come out more wet and clumpy than when you zip them through a food processor.

While you are shredding, preheat your nonstick griddle to high. You want to be able to cook the browns as soon as you're finished prepping the potatoes.

Once your potatoes are all shredded, place them into a vegetable strainer and rinse off any oxidization that has occurred. It does rinse off, believe it or not. Once your potatoes regain their proper color, you can pull out your secret weapon: cheese cloth. Place your shreds into the cloth, wrap them up, and then twist and squeeze every bit of water you can out of the potatoes. The drier the potatoes, the better the browns. Raw potatoes actually have a surprisingly high water content.

Place the shreds in a thin layer on the grill. The thinner the layer, the more successfully they will brown. You can check how well they are browning by lifting up a small section with your spatula. Flip in sections. Toss onto a plate when fully browned, and serve with a condiment of your choice.

Option: Buy frozen hash brown potatoes from your local supermarket (no oil); cook 'em up on your griddle and scarf 'em down.

- -

Breakfast Potato Hash

This recipe will require a bit of planning ahead, as we prefer to use precooked potatoes that have been chilled overnight. Bake them, microwave them, steam them—it doesn't matter. Cook a very large batch so you can use them for other dishes. We're calling this a breakfast meal, but you can eat this for dinner as a main course or serve it as a side dish.

Prep time: 10 minutes; Cook time: 30 minutes
Servings: 2 to 4

1 teaspoon garlic powder
1 teaspoon onion powder
¼ teaspoon powdered rosemary
½ teaspoon salt
¼ teaspoon pepper
2 tablespoons nutritional yeast

4 cooked russet potatoes, refrigerated overnight
1 small onion, peeled and chopped
1 red bell pepper, seeded and chopped
¼ cup low-sodium vegetable broth or water
2 scallions, chopped

Preheat oven to 425 degrees.

Combine dry spices, salt, pepper, and nutritional yeast in a small bowl, and set aside. Cube the cooked potatoes, place in a medium-size bowl. Coat the potatoes with the dry ingredients, and transfer to a cookie sheet. Bake at 425 degrees for 30 minutes.

While the potatoes are baking, sauté the onion and bell pepper at high heat in a wok or large frying pan in the broth or water, until softened. Turn heat to low and simmer. Add more liquid as needed. Once the potatoes are cooked, stir them into the wok or pan and cook at high heat until most of the liquid has been reduced. Top with chopped scallions. Serve with condiment of your choice.

Blueberry I Sigh Bowl

Acai bowls have become a trendy and popular breakfast. The acai comes frozen in packets, which is blended and poured into bowls and usually topped with something crunchy. What you may not know about acai is that it is a fairly high-fat fruit and the frozen packets you find at the grocery might also contain high amounts of processed sugar. Acai bowls are often mixed with guarana, a seed used to power energy drinks and shots. Acai bowls are not as healthy as you might have thought; these are desserts, not meals. So we decided to create a healthy alternative to acai bowls. This recipe uses blended frozen fruit with raw or toasted oats and makes a very appealing breakfast.

Prep time: 5 minutes
Servings: 1

½ cup frozen blueberries
1 small frozen banana
¼ frozen strawberries

¼ cup homemade plant milk

1 tablespoon maple syrup

2 sprigs fresh mint

1 teaspoon lemon juice

½ cup raw or toasted oats

Fresh sliced banana (for garnish)

Add the frozen fruit, plant milk, maple syrup, mint, and lemon juice to a food processor or blender. Blend on high until all ingredients are mixed—you want to keep a fairly thick consistency so try not to overblend. Pour over raw or toasted oats, and top with sliced banana.

- -

Vitamin A+ Muffins

Muffins are a popular breakfast item, and some people believe they are a healthy option. Better a muffin than nothing, right? Well, not so fast. A store-bought muffin can have more fat and sugar than a doughnut. A muffin is really just another word for breakfast cupcake. Do you eat cupcakes for breakfast? Hopefully not! But muffins are such a great size for a quick snack or small breakfast that we came up with a healthier alternative for your skin and the rest of your body.

Prep time: 15 minutes; Cook time: 10 to 12 minutes
Servings: 12 muffins

2½ cups whole wheat white flour (we prefer Bob's Red Mill or
  King Arthur Flour)

2 teaspoons baking powder

¼ teaspoon baking soda

1 teaspoon pumpkin pie spice

¼ cup coconut sugar (or brown sugar)

2 tablespoons maple syrup

2 tablespoons applesauce

¼ cup chickpea flour beaten with ¼ cup water

1½ cup sweet potato purée

Raw oats (optional)

Preheat oven to 375 degrees.

In a large bowl combine the flour, baking powder and soda, pumpkin pie spice, and sugar. In a second large bowl, combine the maple syrup, applesauce, chickpea flour mixture, and potato purée; whisk until completely mixed and smooth.

Pour wet ingredients into dry, fold over with spatula until well blended.

Spoon batter into silicone or nonstick muffin tins. Sprinkle with the optional raw oats; they'll toast and get a bit crispy while you bake.

Bake for 10 to 12 minutes. Muffins should be somewhat brown; do not overcook. Test muffin with toothpick. If it comes out clean, they're done.

Allow pan to cool for 5 to 10 minutes before you try to remove the muffins. Top with jam, and then jam!

- -

Happy Halloween Pumpkin Muffins

Every time you can find a way to get some pumpkin into your body, you are doing your skin a big favor. A cup of pumpkin is loaded with 197 percent of the RDA for vitamin A. Yes, 197 percent! Vitamin A is a known anti-inflammatory agent and is a powerful tool in your acne arsenal. So chow down on these muffins as often as you like: they are not just good tasting, they are good for you.

> 2 cups gluten-free flour mix
> ½ cup old-fashioned rolled oats
> ½ teaspoon xanthan gum
> ¾ cup raw sugar
> 2½ teaspoons baking powder
> ½ teaspoon baking soda
> 1 teaspoon pumpkin pie spice
> ½ cup raisins
> 1 cup rice milk
> ½ cup boiling water
> ½ cup canned pumpkin purée
> ¼ cup applesauce
> 1 tablespoon lemon juice

Preheat oven to 350 degrees.

In a medium bowl, combine the flour, oats, xantham gum, sugar, baking powder and soda, spice, and raisins. In a second bowl, whisk the milk, water, purée, applesauce, and lemon juice together.

Make a hole in the middle of the dry mixture. Pour the wet ingredients into the hole. Gently start folding dry ingredients into wet, until completely combined.

Fill each cup in a nonstick muffin pan about two-thirds full. Bake for 20 to 25 minutes, or until a toothpick comes out clean. Let cool before eating—but these muffins are particularly good while still warm, with strawberry jam on top. Toss in your gym bag for a quick source of energy while you're working out.

Ooh La La French Toast

The basic recipe for French toast has been around for a couple of thousand years. It's essentially bread dipped in eggs and milk and fried. Vegan versions usually involve tofu. We're not including eggs, dairy, or tofu in our version of French toast, but we are frying the bread— just not in gallons of butter or oil. Your skin says, "Thank you."

Prep time: 10 minutes; Cook time: 3 to 5 minutes
Servings: 2 to 4

⅛ cup chickpea flour beaten with ⅛ cup water
2 teaspoons maple syrup
1 cup homemade plant milk
¼ teaspoon cinnamon
1 teaspoon vanilla extract
1 loaf crusty whole wheat bread (unsliced), preferably a day
  old
Fresh fruit
Maple syrup

Preheat a griddle to a high heat. Thoroughly mix all ingredients, except for the bread, in a large shallow bowl. Chill in the refrigerator for about 30 minutes.

Slice the bread into four thick pieces. Dip the bread in the batter until soaked on both sides. Place on the griddle; cook until golden-brown on one side, and then flip. Top with fruit of choice and maple syrup.

- -

Polenta Fiesta Scramble

This breakfast is for those who enjoy Mexican-style omelets or scrambled eggs. We've never actually eaten eggs ourselves but wanted to create a lower-fat alternative that egg lovers and plant-based eaters could all enjoy. Don't forget to try this quick and easy breakfast for lunch and dinner (stuff it in a wrap for lunch or use it for Taco Tuesdays for dinner). The smell will drive you crazy while it's cooking; it's so dang good.

Prep time: 10 minutes; Cook time: 30 minutes
Servings: 6

1 red bell pepper, chopped
4-ounce can diced green chiles
2 tablespoons vegetable broth
1 8-ounce package sliced mushrooms
2 teaspoons garlic powder
½ teaspoon chili powder
⅛ tsp dried oregano
½ teaspoon smoked paprika
1 16-ounce tube precooked polenta
2 tablespoons salsa (for garnish)
Onion (for garnish)
Black beans (for garnish)

Sauté pepper and chiles in the veggie broth; add more broth as needed. Add mushrooms and spices, and stir until softened. Slice polenta into about 1/2-inch rounds, and crumble carefully into mix. Do not over-mix; allow the polenta to cook enough to retain some of its texture. Garnish with salsa, onions, or black beans.

HANDHELDS: WRAPS, BURRITOS, AND SANDWICHES

Some people might like to refer to wraps, burritos, and sandwiches as "lunch," perhaps because of their easy portability. Virtually every culture on the planet feasts on some sort of sandwich, burrito, or hand pie. Whether sold by a street vendor in Mumbai or a fast-food burger joint in Los Angeles, handheld meals are popular because they are easy to eat when you're on the run. Pop them in a paper bag or backpack, and your meal goes where you go. We hesitate to call our handhelds lunch, however, because we want to encourage you to devour them anytime of the day or night.

- -

Mushroom Bun Me

This handheld might just become your new favorite "lunch" (or whatever). This is our version of the traditional Vietnamese *bánh mì* sandwich. *Bánh mì* is the fortunate result of blending French and Vietnamese cuisine. From the French, we get crunchy baguettes and paté; from the Vietnamese, coriander, carrots, and daikon. Vietnamese baguettes are lighter than their French counterparts and are usually made without oil or shortening. If there is a Vietnamese store or bakery in your community, buy a bag of baguettes for your sandwich, freezing what you don't immediately use.

Our *bánh mì* replaces meat with mushrooms and mayonnaise with anything but mayo—mustard, homemade hummus, or whatever you fancy. Bundle this baby up in paper and have a picnic in the park—if you can prevent yourself from eating it before you get out the door, that is.

Prep time: 10 minutes; Cook time: 2 to 3 minutes
Servings: 1 to 2

¼ cup shredded carrot
¼ cup shredded daikon radish
½ cup rice wine vinegar

1 8-ounce package sliced mushrooms
2 tablespoons tamari, soy sauce, or
  Bragg Liquid Aminos
Vietnamese baguette (or oil-free French baguette,
  ciabatta, or submarine sandwich roll)
1 small sliced cucumber
¼ cup sliced onion
2 tablespoons sliced pepperoncini
Bunch of fresh cilantro
1 teaspoon pepper
lime juice (optional)

Shred carrot and radish with food processor or cheese grater. Place carrots and radishes in a mason jar, and add vinegar and 1/4 cup water. Shake, and allow to pickle overnight.

When it's time to make your sandwich, cook the mushrooms in tamari and 2 tablespoons water for 2 to 3 minutes, until slightly soft. Slice your baguette in half, and pile with pickled mixture, sliced cucumber, sliced onions, mushrooms, and pepperoncini. Sprinkle with pepper and drizzle with lime juice. Hungry yet?

Option: Substitute roasted eggplant, jackfruit, or roasted beets for the mushrooms (but mushrooms are the best).

- -

Chicka-boom Curry Sandwich

We love chickpeas, curry, India relish, and thick whole wheat bread. So why not have them all at the same time? You can use the chickpea mixture on a sandwich, with a bowl, or roll it up into a lettuce leaf. Double or triple the batch and have "lunch" ready for a few days in advance.

1 can chickpeas drained (reserve liquid)
2 stalks celery, chopped
2 green onions, thinly sliced
½ small white onion, chopped
2 garlic cloves, minced
2 tablespoons stone-ground mustard
2 teaspoons yellow mustard

1 tablespoon sugarcane vinegar
  (or rice wine, if sugarcane is not available)
1 tablespoon curry powder
1 tablespoon India relish
Sandwich bread (oil-free) of your choice
Shredded carrots, sprouts, and tomatoes, for toppings

Smash chickpeas with potato masher. Stir in remaining ingredients until mixed. Scoop onto bread, add toppings, and gobble it up.

Option: Thin mixture with lemon juice and reserved bean water and use as veggie dip.

- -

Gimme Potpies

One of the top requests from our readers and viewers are quick and easy ideas for a home-packed lunch. We tell them to pack rice and beans in a microwaveable bowl—and they say give us pie. So here's the pie! These lunch boxes freeze well, so you can make a double or triple batch and reheat them in a microwave at work or school.

Prep time: 15 minutes; Cook time: 25 to 30 minutes
Servings: About six potpies

Crust
3 cups gluten-free flour mix
1½ teaspoons salt
1 teaspoon xanthum gum
1 teaspoon baking powder
⅔ cup applesauce
⅔ cup ice water
1 teaspoon apple cider vinegar

Filling
½ cup chopped onion
2 cups low-sodium vegetable broth or water
½ teaspoon paprika
1 teaspoon dried thyme

¼ cup gluten-free flour mix
½ cup rice milk
3 carrots, chopped
½ cup frozen peas
½ cup frozen corn
1 cup peeled, chopped, and precooked potato

For the crust: Preheat oven to 350 degrees.

Whisk together flour, salt, xanthun gum, and baking powder until completely blended. Add applesauce and stir until it is mixed into flour. Pour ice water in slowly, blending as you add, to get the right consistency. You want sticky but not slimy. Knead into smooth dough.

Cover and chill in the refrigerator for at least 30 minutes. The dough will roll more easily if it is cold.

For the filling: While the dough is chilling, prepare your filling. Sauté onions in water or vegetable broth for about five minutes or until softened. Add spices and flour, and whisk with fork until thickened. Add rice milk and broth, and then carrots, peas, corn, and potatoes. Bring to a boil, and simmer on low heat for about 10 minutes, or until the carrots are softened.

For the pies: Tear off the dough in pieces, and roll out between two sheets of parchment paper to about 3 inches in diameter, 1/4 inch thick. Arrange the dough in a nonstick muffin tin to form bottom crust. Fill the bottom crust, and top with another piece of dough. Seal the edges by pinching with fingers. Pierce the top lightly with a fork to vent.

Bake for about 25 minutes, or until the crust has browned.

- -

Nina's Lentil Femwich

The traditional sloppy Joe is made with oil and meat and fried. This healthy, inexpensive plant-based version is one of our favorites to serve when we have guests because it takes almost no time to prepare and cook, and everyone consumes it like they're getting a special treat. (Not a manwich, but guys do love to eat them too!) The leftovers are even better the next day.

> *Prep time: 10 minutes; Cook time: 40 minutes (Instant Pot), about 1 hour (stovetop)*
> *Servings: 8*

1 red bell pepper, chopped
1 green bell pepper, chopped
½ cup dried minced onions
1 teaspoon chili powder
1 cooked russet potato, mashed with skin
3 cups dry green lentils
4 cups low-sodium vegetable broth or water (about 1 carton)
2 cups ketchup (no high-fructose corn syrup)
½ cup rice wine vinegar

Preparation with Instant Pot: Add all ingredients to an Instant Pot or other electric pressure cooker, and set timer for 30 minutes.

Preparation on stovetop: Add all ingredients to large pot, bring to a boil on high. Lower heat, and simmer covered for about 1 hour (occasionally stirring to make sure the lentils do not burn or stick).

Serve on your favorite whole wheat bun with lettuce and BBQ sauce, or on brown rice.

- -

KISS Burrito

Does anyone really need to be told how to make a burrito? You take a tortilla, fill it with things you like, and roll it up. That's our big, exciting, groundbreaking burrito recipe. But seriously, folks, we'll take you by the hand and break this whole burrito thing down slowly to you. Burritos are life!

Whole wheat fat-free tortilla
Rice
Beans

Lettuce

Tomatoes

Salsa

We're not providing measurements because only you can determine how *gordito* you want your burrito. Add ingredients to the tortilla in this order, and then roll your tortilla.

Now that you have learned how to properly prepare a KISS burrito, let's get into the variations. Here are some items that add some zing to the classic burrito: frozen roasted corn, steamed broccoli, steamed squash, the pickled mixture from Mushroom Bun Me (see page 195), sprouts, sliced mushrooms. Use mashed potatoes instead of rice, and toast the burrito in an oven or toaster oven until the tortilla is brown and crispy. Yes, we did say mashed potatoes in the burrito. Don't laugh until you've tried it!

- -

Spot the Carrot Dog

This quickie recipe is inspired by our friend Ann Esselstyn, coauthor of *Prevent and Reverse Heart Disease Cookbook*. Ann is a wonderfully inventive cook—she makes healthy taste heavenly. This "hot dog" featuring a big carrot is both skin and smile friendly. Who doesn't love hot dogs! (Hopefully not you, the traditional ones anyway, as they're full of fat- and cancer-promoting preservatives.) The trick to this lies in the condiments.

Prep time: 10 minutes; Cook time: About 10 minutes
Servings: 1 to 2

1 large carrot, peeled (or more, depending on how many dogs
    you're producing)
1 whole wheat hot dog bun
Condiment of choice: ketchup, mustard, relish, and so on

Steam the carrot in a pressure cooker for about 1 minute. The carrot can be boiled, if you prefer, but it takes forever to boil a whole carrot. Toast the bun. Add "dog" to bun and top with condiments.

Option: Top with the pickled mixture from Mushroom Bun Me (page 195)—because it's great on just about anything.

Samosa Hermosa

A samosa is a fried or baked pastry, usually stuffed with spicy meat, vegetables, or potatoes. The samosa originated in Central Asia but has made its way around the whole planet. They're often vegan and usually delicious—and almost always loaded with fat. We've named our version Samosa Hermosa, as we are using fat-free tortillas instead of pastry, and no frying or oil is involved.

Prep time: 10 minutes; Cook time: 15 minutes
Servings: 2 to 4

Fat-free whole wheat tortillas

Filling
2 cups mashed potatoes (freshly prepared, or leftovers)
½ cup frozen or fresh peas
½ white onion, chopped
1 teaspoon garlic powder
2 teaspoons curry
1 teaspoon garam masala spice
1 teaspoon chili power
3 tablespoons fresh coriander, chopped
2 tablespoons lemon juice

Combine all the filling ingredients in a microwaveable glass bowl. Heat in the microwave for about 4 minutes. Remove, stir, and set aside.

Heat the tortillas in the microwave for about 30 seconds, until softened. Remove the tortillas, set on a plate, and scoop filling onto tortillas.

Fold each tortilla into a triangle shape, securing the ends with a small amount of water. Lightly spritz each tortilla with water; this will help it crisp without oil.

We like to toast these singly in a toaster oven for about five minutes, but if you are making several, then baking is more practical.

Preheat oven to 450 degrees, and bake on a cookie sheet for 5 to 10 minutes, or until the tortillas are crispy brown.

Serve with chutney, mustard, or ketchup. Stonewall Kitchen makes several very good chutneys, most of which are clear skin compliant.

Get in My Belly Burgers

This recipe is a variation of the classic bean burgers developed by our friend Jeff Novick, who is also a trained chef and registered dietician. We learned how to make burgers from Chef Jeff when we were only fifteen years old, while shooting the *Fast Food* DVD series with him. Very few chefs are also dieticians, which makes Jeff unusual—he's also a brilliant researcher, who helped us a lot while we were working on this book. So please give a round of applause to Mr. Novick for inspiring this recipe, and then pat yourself on the back for making these burgers yourself!

Prep time: 10 minutes; Cook time: About 5 minutes
Servings: 12 burgers

1 cup cooked beans of choice, chilled overnight
½ cup cooked barley, chilled overnight
1 cup cooked lentils, chilled overnight
½ cooked brown rice, chilled overnight
½ cup oats
¼ cup ketchup or BBQ sauce
½ cup dried onions
1 tablespoon poultry seasoning
Whole wheat burger buns
Lettuce
Tomatoes
Sweet red onion
Pickles
Condiments of choice

We are asking you to chill the beans, barley, lentils, and rice over-night, as the mash binds together better with cold ingredients. In a large bowl, mash beans, barley, lentils, rice, oats, and ketchup or BBQ sauce together with a potato masher. Add more sauce if the mixture is too dry. Use a masher, not a food processor, because you want burgers—not a spread.

Add the onions and poultry seasoning and squish together with fingers. (Squish is the most accurate way to describe how you mix these burgers!) Form into patties, and place them on a cookie sheet. We like to chill the burgers for at least an hour before cooking, giving the flavors and mix a chance to set.

Preheat a grill (we use a Cuisinart panini grill). Grill the patties for about 5 minutes, until heated through or slightly crispy. Toast your bun, add your lettuce, tomatoes, pickles, onions, and condiments—and it's Burger Time!

> Option: For some variety in your burgers, you can replace rice with one of the following: ½ cup sweet potatoes (add 1 table-spoon curry), ½ cup mashed potatoes, ½ cup mashed cauliflower, or 1 cup minced mushrooms.

SOUPS

Let's just get this out of the way. Soup is not just "good food"; soup is good *skin* food. Not only is it supremely delicious and filling, it is also highly nutritious (vegetables cooked into soup retain more of their nutrients). Tomatoes, for example, are bursting with lycopene, which is made more bioavailable when cooked in a soup. Lycopene helps protect against skin damage caused by the sun, among its many other virtues. They also impart tremendous flavor, as well as health, to the broth. Adding carrots to your soup increases the bioavailability of beta-carotene as well, as the cell walls of those tough little roots are broken down by the heat. Beta-carotene also helps to repair skin tissue. When your soup includes starches like rice, potatoes, or barley along with your veggies, you have everything your body requires to power itself through a long day or a cold night. We hope you start thinking of soup not just as the start of your lunch or dinner but as the alpha and the omega—aka the beginning, middle, and end—of your meal.

Many of our soup and chili recipes use what the French call mirepoix as a base. Mirepoix consists of onions, carrots, and celery. With these three talented veggies in the mix, your veggie soup possibilities are endless. As you gain confidence in your kitchen, remember mirepoix. Your soup pot will do the happy dance on your stove if you do, guaranteed.

- -

Mom's PC Black Bean Chili

As you may have guessed, this is one of our mother's recipes. And by PC we don't mean politically correct, we mean pressure cooker. Our mom developed this recipe expressly for the pressure cooker, so she would be able to feed us a hearty meal and fast. We grew up eating this chili. While this chili was warm and wonderful on one of our few chilly Southern California days, we ate this pretty much year-round. It's terrific served over rice, french fries, baked potatoes, corn bread, or on its own sprinkled with a bit of nutritional yeast. This chili is our kind of comfort food.

Prep time: 15 minutes; Cook time: 80 minutes (Instant Pot)
Servings: 6 to 8

2 cups dried black beans
1 to 2 onions, coarsely chopped
1 to 2 teaspoons minced garlic
1 large red bell pepper, seeded and chopped
2 celery stalks, chopped
1 to 2 carrots, chopped
1 to 2 dried chipotle peppers, seeded and chopped
2 tablespoons chili powder
1 28-ounce can diced fire-roasted tomatoes
1 32-ounce carton low-sodium vegetable broth
½ cup dry green lentils
1 cup frozen roasted corn

Add all ingredients to a pressure cooker, and cook for 80 minutes

Purée about 1 cup of the chili in a blender and return to the pressure cooker. Mix well and serve. Season with a splash of tamari (soy sauce), if desired. It's nearly mandatory to eat this chili with cornbread; luckily there is a recipe available on page 230.

- -

Creamy Potato Power Chowder

Hot, cold, windy, rainy...today is the perfect day for soup! Why not get a little adventurous and have this soup for breakfast?

Prep time: 10 minutes; Cook time: 30 minutes (Instant Pot),
  about 70 minutes (stovetop)
Servings: 6

6 Yukon Gold potatoes, cubed (no need to peel)
4 stalks celery, chopped
2 carrots, cubed
½ cup dried minced onions
2 teaspoons garlic powder
4 cups low-sodium vegetable broth or water
  (about 1 carton)
1 cup nondairy milk of choice
2 teaspoons poultry seasoning
2 cups fresh or frozen corn
1 tablespoon nutritional yeast

Preparation with Instant pot: Add all ingredients except for the corn to an Instant Pot or other electric pressure cooker; set the timer for 30 minutes. Once the pressure has been released and the lid has been removed, the soup can be blended with an immersion blender.

After the soup is blended, add the corn and return the lid to the pot. Let it sit for a couple of minutes, without adding additional heat. The corn will be warmed by the hot soup.

Preparation on stovetop: Add all the ingredients except for the corn to a pot; bring to boil on high. Reduce heat to medium, and simmer covered for about 1 hour, until the potatoes are softened.

Remove the soup from the stove, and use an immersion blender to cream the soup. Once the soup is blended, add the corn and return the lid to the pot. Let it sit for a couple of minutes, without adding additional heat. The corn will be warmed by the hot soup.

Option: Top with Smoky Roasted Mushrooms (recipe below).

- -

Smoky Roasted Mushrooms

A scrumptious topping for soups or baked potato—bacon flavor!

Prep time: 30 minutes; Cook time: 30 minutes
Servings: 2 to 4

1 8-ounce package of mushroom of choice (sliced are great,
    save on that prep time)
2 tablespoons tamari, soy sauce, or Bragg Liquid Aminos
1 tablespoon maple syrup
¾ teaspoon liquid smoke
½ teaspoon smoked paprika
1 garlic clove, crushed

Preheat oven to 400 degrees.

Quickly whisk all the ingredients, except the mushrooms, in a bowl. Add sliced mushrooms to the bowl, and cover the mushrooms completely with the marinade. Let the marinade sit for about 30 minutes.

Transfer mushrooms to a cookie sheet protected by a silicone liner. Roast for about 30 minutes.

- -

Freezer Soup

This is another of our mom's specialties. And no, we're not telling you to eat soup-sicles. Freezer soup is one of those dishes that is never prepared the same way twice because the ingredients consist of basically whatever you have in your freezer and/or leftover in the fridge. Below are potential ingredients for your own freezer soup. Measuring is optional, and the freezer gets to decide what makes an appearance in the pot.

Prep time: 5 minutes; Cook time: 30 minutes
Servings: 4 to 6

1 cup frozen corn

1 cup frozen peas

1 cup frozen edamame

1 cup frozen kale

1 cup leftover beans

1 cup leftover rice

½ cup dry green lentils

4 cups low-sodium vegetable broth (about 1 carton)

2 tablespoons poultry seasoning

Place all the ingredients into an Instant Pot or other electric pressure cooker, along with 4 cups of water, and cook for 30 minutes. Thank your lucky stars that you were smart enough to stock your freezer with a bunch of cool vegetables (pun intended), when you have to scrape together a quickie meal in a pinch. This is another reminder to cook rice and beans in bulk, so you can throw something together anytime, day or night.

- -

Golden Sunrise Split Pea Soup

Does this name imply that we're trying to convince you to eat soup for breakfast, again? That's not a bad idea, but this soup actually reminds us of the vibrant colors you'll find in a perfect sunrise. And you'll also find them in this soup!

Prep time: 10 minutes; Cook time: 30 minutes
Servings: 4 to 6

2 cups yellow split peas, rinsed

1 brown onion, chopped

4 garlic cloves, crushed

2 teaspoons ginger powder

2 tablespoons curry powder

4 cups low-sodium vegetable broth (about 1 carton)

2 cups coconut water

2 cups roasted and chopped sweet potatoes

1 cup finely chopped fresh kale
Chopped green onions (optional garnish)
Minced parsley (optional garnish)

Again, we recommend using a pressure cooker so your beautiful soup will be available to you in about a half hour. Put all the ingredients except for the kale into the pressure cooker. Set the timer for 30 minutes. Once the soup is cooked, add fresh kale and stir. Don't cook the kale with the soup; the heat of the cooked soup softens it sufficiently. Garnish with optional chopped green onions and/or parsley.

- -

Gratitude Butternut Squash Bisque

The butternut is a winter squash, similar in taste and texture to pumpkin. Like the pumpkin, it's also rich with vitamin A, as well as vitamins C and E. This is a highly skin-friendly fruit (yes, it's actually a fruit!). Our family serves this dish at Thanksgiving, hence the name. We tend to eat this seasonally with fresh butternuts, but if you can't wait until autumn, many Costco stores sell frozen butternut chunks year-round. If you choose to use fresh butternut, be sure to peel it with a squash peeler. Your peeling time will be shortened considerably, and you can get on with the fun of cleaning out seeds. Actually it's not that fun, but this soup is worth the effort.

Prep time: 15 minutes; Cook time: 30 minutes
Servings: 4 to 6

1 whole butternut squash, peeled and chopped into chunks
  (or 2-pound bag of Costco frozen squash)
l large russet potato, peeled and chopped into chunks
2 large carrots, peeled and chopped into chunks
2 cups coconut water
4 cups low-sodium vegetable broth
  (about 1 carton)
2 tablespoons maple syrup
1 teaspoon ground cinnamon
½ teaspoon ground nutmeg

Add all the ingredients to an Instant Pot or other electric pressure cooker. Set time for 30 minutes. Once the pressure has been released, blend the soup in the pot with an immersion blender. Transfer to a pretty soup tureen, and you're ready to celebrate.

- -

Valley Berbere Lentil Stew

This recipe is inspired by the red lentil stew our mother used to make for our brother Willie. We say she made it for him because he would basically just eat a whole pot by himself. And we're from the Valley, hence "Valley Stew." We've incorporated a few of our own favorites to Mom's basic recipe, like skin-friendly sweet potatoes. *Berbere* spice is a staple of Ethiopian cuisine and includes chile peppers, garlic, ginger, basil, *korarima*, rue, *ajwain*, and more. *Berbere* can be hot, so add more or less, depending on how much heat you enjoy. Willie can tolerate a lot more *berbere* spice than we can!

Prep time: 10 minutes; Cook time: 30 minutes
Servings: 4 to 6

1 cup chopped onion
2 tablespoons berbere spice mixture
2 garlic cloves, minced
4 cups low-sodium vegetable broth (approximately 1 carton)
2 cups dry red lentils
1 large russet potato, peeled and chopped
2 large red yams, peeled and chopped
1 24-ounce jar oil-free, low-sodium pasta sauce
1 tablespoon ground fresh ginger

Add all ingredients along with 1 cup water to an Instant Pot or other electric pressure cooker. (It's easy to burn red lentils on a stovetop, so we recommend only using a pressure cooker for this dish.) Cook for 30 minutes. Stir stew thoroughly once the pot is opened to blend ingredients. You can eat this stew chunky style or use an immersion blender to create a more creamy consistency. This stew is a filling stand-alone meal, and it's also excellent over rice.

Mushroom Mania Lentil and Barley Stew

This recipe calls for three different types of mushrooms. Why? Well, because we love mushrooms, of course! Crimini are baby portobello mushrooms and are just easier to slice and chop for soups than their grown counterparts. Use the big guys if the crimini are not available at your grocery. If you don't have access to dried shitakes or crimini mushrooms, you can replace with an additional pound of button mushrooms. This is most definitely a mushroom soup. Some people prefer a starchier soup, so add more barley if that's you. A half a cup of barley goes a long way, though.

Prep time: 30 minutes; Cook time: 30 minutes
Servings: 4 to 6

1 large yellow onion, chopped
½ cup chopped celery,
½ cup carrots, peeled and chopped
2 garlic cloves, crushed
1 pound white button mushrooms sliced
½ pound crimini mushrooms, sliced
8 dried shitake mushrooms, chopped
  (soak for 20 minutes in boiling water and
  discard stems)
½ cup pearl barley
½ cup dry green lentils
2 bay leaves
½ teaspoon powdered rosemary
6 dried shitake mushrooms
4 cups low-sodium vegetable or
  mushroom broth

Add all the ingredients to an Instant Pot or other electric pressure cooker along with 4 cups water. Cook for 30 minutes. If you have left-over cooked rice, you can use a cup of rice instead of the barley. When the rice is cooked twice, it behaves remarkably like barley in a soup.

Blessed Broccoli and Cauliflower Bisque Soup

Creamy bisque soups like this oftentimes contain large quantities of dairy and/or chicken-based broth. Ours gets its creaminess from potato starch and an immersion blender. This is a "blessed" soup as it contains both broccoli and cauliflower—superstar veggies for your skin. Broccoli and cauliflower are members of the mustard family. The part of the plant you eat is actually their flower buds; cauliflower is a flower. They contain glucoraphanin, a compound unique to these two plants. Glucoraphanin helps to regenerate damaged skin, so this soup is beneficial to your healing process. It's also delectable and simple to make.

Prep time: 10 minutes; Cook time: 25 minutes
Servings: 4 to 6

2 leeks, chopped
2 stalks celery, chopped
4 garlic cloves, crushed
1 head broccoli florets or 1 pound frozen
1 head cauliflower florets or 1 pound frozen
6 large Yukon Gold potatoes, cubed
  (no need to peel)
½ cup fresh or frozen kale, chopped
½ cup homemade plant milk
4 cups low-sodium vegetable broth
  (about 1 carton)
1 tablespoon poultry seasoning
Salt and pepper, to taste

Add all ingredients to an Instant Pot or other electric pressure cooker. Cook for 25 minutes. After pressure is released, blend the soup with an immersion blender until creamy. Add water to thin the soup, if necessary. This soup is actually quite good cold, as well. Chilled overnight the flavors have a chance to really blend. It's kind of like a broccoli smoothie.

Dill-icious Cold Cucumber Soup

We love fresh herbs, and of course we love soup. But we also are native Southern California girls, and it can get hot here during the summer. This soup is for those times when you crave the filling-ness (is that a new word?!) of soup but don't want the heat. This is a great quickie summer soup as it doesn't require cooking. Fresh herbs are preferred, by the way.

Prep time: 10 minutes; Chill time: 2 hours
Servings: 4 to 6

3 cups low-sodium vegetable broth
4 Yukon Gold potatoes, precooked, chilled, and cubed
  (no need to peel)
6 Persian cucumbers, peeled and seeded, or one
  English cucumber, peeled and seeded
½ cup sweet red onion
2 celery stalks, chopped
½ cup fresh dill
¼ cup fresh parsley
¼ cup fresh basil
½ cup fresh arugula
1 teaspoon dried thyme
½ teaspoon rosemary powder
2 green onions, thinly chopped

Add all the ingredients to a food processor or blender, and blend until smooth. Add water in increments, if necessary, to thin the soup. Allow to chill for at least 2 hours, preferably overnight. Garnish with green onions.

Say Cheez Creamy Cauliflower Soup

Have you ever heard of the "don't eat white foods diet"? Well, we totally disagree with that scheme, as it would mean forsaking fantastic foods like cauliflower and potatoes. They are both highly skin-friendly veggies, and potatoes are satiating. Eat these white foods—especially in this cheezy but no-cheese soup.

Prep time: 15 minutes; Cook time: 25 minutes
Servings: 4 to 6

1 small white onion, chopped
1 cauliflower, cut into florets
4 Yukon Gold potatoes, cubed (no need to peel)
2 garlic cloves, crushed
2 stalks celery, chopped
1 large carrot, peeled and chopped
6 cups low-sodium vegetable broth
2 teaspoons smoked paprika
1 tablespoon poultry seasoning
½ cup nutritional yeast
¼ cup yellow mustard
½ cup all-purpose flour
2 teaspoons arrowroot powder
2 cups homemade plant milk or veggie broth
Salt and pepper to taste

Add all the ingredients to an Instant Pot or other electric pressure cooker, and cook for 25 minutes. Blend with an immersion blender in the pot until smooth. Serve with a crunchy loaf of French bread. Don't be afraid to dip!

BOWLS

What is a bowl, exactly? Other than something you eat out of? Bowls have gained popularity in recent years, usually called Buddha bowls. Bowls typically consist of a starch, a vegetable, a legume, and maybe some raw greens. Does that sound like a fancy term for a salad? (You might note that we are not including salad recipes in this book because do you really need a recipe for salad? And vegans don't eat just salads, anyway.) We kind of feel the same way about bowls. So rather than waste your time with twenty different bowl recipes you are probably never going to eat or use, we are going to tell you how to build your own bowl. We like to use the classic white nine-inch bowls for this one-dish meal. The nine-inch bowls hold a lot of food, and they look pretty on Instagram.

Clear Skin Diet Bowl or Buddha Bowl

Prep time: 5 minutes; Cook time: 15 minutes
Servings: 1

Potatoes, brown rice, or pasta
Vegetable of choice
Legume of choice
Kale, spinach, or romaine (what do you feel like?)

Add to bowl, top with condiment of choice, and eat.

MAIN DISHES, ENTRÉES, CASSEROLES

To be honest, we think just about everything in this book could be a main dish. Again, if it's good for dinner, it's also good for breakfast or lunch. If you eat leftover Macky Cheez for breakfast, does that mean it's not a main dish anymore? That said, we understand that people can get caught up in traditional food terminology, which is why we added these particular dishes to this section. If you make enchiladas for dinner, pack them for school or lunch the next day. That's the beauty of cooking in bulk—leftover is just another way of saying "future meal."

KISS Baked Potato

Is a baked potato a main dish? In our house it is. We've tried just about every method out there to cook a potato, and this is our favorite.

Prep time: 1 minute; Cook time: 75 minutes

Servings: 1 potato equals 1 serving
1 to 8 russet potatoes or
1 to 8 sweet potatoes

Preheat oven to 425 degrees. Poke potato(es) several times with a knife. Wrap in parchment paper and then aluminum foil. Bake for 75 minutes.

> Option: Crispy steak fries! Chill potatoes in aluminum foil overnight. Remove from foil, cut into steak fries, and bake on a cookie sheet at 425 degrees for 35 minutes. These fries make a great snack, side dish, or travel companion.

Macky Cheez

"Oh, I just can't give up cheese." How many times have we heard people say that when confronted with the idea of going totally vegan? A million? It's actually not the dairy that people crave, it's the sour, creamy texture they adore. Because we want you to feel totally comfortable and happy transitioning to a dairy-free lifestyle, we came up with this healthy alternative to the traditional macaroni and cheese casserole. You may want to double or triple this recipe, because it's *so darn good*. We are using rice pasta for this recipe because the rice pasta itself is very creamy and satisfying.

Prep time: 15 minutes; Cook time: 40 minutes
Servings: 2 to 4

1 box rice pasta
1 head of broccoli, cut into florets
1 cup frozen corn
½ pound sliced mushrooms
2 Yukon Gold potatoes, cubed (no need to peel)
½ cup rice milk (optional)
½ cup low-sodium vegetable broth
2 tablespoons flour
3 tablespoons nutritional yeast flakes
1 tablespoon yellow mustard
1 4-ounce jar roasted red bell peppers (in water), drained
1 teaspoon garlic powder
1 teaspoon onion powder

Preheat oven to 375 degrees.

Steam the potatoes until tender (about 20 minutes in a pressure cooker, 30 minutes on the stove). Cook the pasta as directed; drain and return to the pot. Add broccoli florets, frozen corn, and mushrooms to the pasta and cover. The heat of the pasta will warm the veggies while still retaining some crunch. Add cooked potatoes, rice milk, broth, flour, nutritional yeast, peppers, garlic and onion powder, and mustard to blender. Blend until completely combined.

Pour the sauce from the blender onto the pasta and stir. Transfer the pasta to a casserole pan. Bake for 40 minutes at 375 degrees. Add salt or soy sauce to taste, if you feel like you need it.

- -

Sweet Potato Pizza Crust with Roasted Veggies

A pizza crust made with...sweet potatoes? Well, that's an interesting idea. Don't be scared; give it a try. You will be pleasantly surprised at how a pizza packed with your favorite skin vitamin, vitamin A, can be.

Prep time: 20 minutes; Cook time: 40 minutes
Servings: 2 to 4

Crust
6 cups peeled and cubed sweet potatoes
2 cups gluten-free flour mix
1 tablespoon applesauce
1 tablespoon rice wine vinegar
1 teaspoon dried basil
1 teaspoon dried oregano
1 teaspoon dried garlic powder
1 teaspoon dried onion powder
Toppings
1 24-ounce jar oil-free, sodium-free tomato or pizza sauce
1 bag frozen artichokes (thawed)
½ head broccoli, chopped into florets
1 cup sliced cherry tomatoes
8 ounces sliced mushrooms
4 garlic cloves, crushed

½ cup arugula, shredded
½ cup spinach, shredded
Chopped fresh green bell peppers (optional garnish)
Nutritional yeast (optional garnish)

Preheat oven to 400 degrees.

Steam the sweet potatoes for about 10 minutes in the pressure cooker, or 25 minutes on the stovetop. Once the potatoes are very soft, transfer to a large mixing bowl and mash thoroughly. Add in the remainder of the crust ingredients along with 3 tablespoons water and blend completely.

Scoop the mixture onto parchment paper on a pizza stone and spread into circle. You will want to get the mixture to about 1/3 inch. Bake for about 30 minutes, or until the crust is browned and firm. Let cool before you add toppings.

Once your crust has cooled, arrange your toppings and bake for another 5 to 10 minutes. Keep an eye on the greens because they can burn easily. Once your pizza is out of the oven, sprinkle with optional peppers or nutritional yeast for some extra zing.

- -

Lazy Lentil Loaf

Why lazy? Because you can spend about five minutes or less preparing an entrée for dinner, and then have plenty of time to read a book or check on your social media empire. Nina's Femwich filling (see page 198) is one of those recipes to make in bulk because you can use it as the basis for several other meals. This loaf makes a surprisingly delicious and satisfying main course. Serve with one of our soup or bowl recipes.

Prep time: 5 or fewer minutes; Cook time: 50 minutes
Servings: 4 to 6

For loaf
3 cups Femwich filling, chilled
½ cup uncooked oats
1 cup cooked brown rice
½ cup cooked barley

For glaze

3 tablespoons ketchup

1 tablespoon rice wine vinegar

1 tablespoon maple syrup

Preheat oven to 350 degrees.

Add the three cups of Femwich filling mix to a bowl, and mash with potato masher. Add oats, rice, and barley, and mash thoroughly. Transfer mixture to a loaf pan.

For glaze, whisk together ketchup, vinegar, and maple syrup until blended. Drizzle onto the loaf.

Bake for 40 to 50 minutes. Let cool slightly before serving. Pair with mashed potatoes and gravy.

I Like It Like That Lasagna

Why do we "like it like that"? Because this lasagna is easy, healthy, filling, and skin friendly. Who wouldn't like it like that!

Prep time: 15 minutes; Cook time: 1 hour
Servings: 2 to 4

Cheezy sauce (use Macky Cheese sauce on page 215)

3 large sweet potatoes, preroasted and peeled

1 pound package lasagna noodles

1 pound crimini or portobello mushrooms, thinly sliced

2 garlic cloves, crushed

1 pound frozen spinach, thawed and liquid squeezed out

1 fresh zucchini, thinly sliced

1 fresh yellow squash, thinly sliced

½ cup fresh basil, minced

1 to 2 24-ounce jars oil-free, low-sodium pasta sauce

Preheat oven to 350 degrees.

Make the cheezy sauce. Mash the sweet potatoes in a separate bowl. Spread a thin layer of the sauce, followed by the sweet potatoes, onto the bottom of a 13 x 9-inch glass baking dish. Layer with uncooked lasagna noodles, Macky Cheez sauce, garlic and vegetables. Reserve about 1/2 cup of the cheez sauce.

Cover the pan with foil, and bake for 45 minutes. Uncover, use remainder of cheez sauce, and continue baking for another 15 minutes, or until the top is somewhat browned.

Remove from the oven, and let stand for at least 15 minutes before you cut the noodles. This recipe is even better the next day. Can you say "lunch"?

Quickie Cauliflower Curry

The red lentils and curry lend this recipe its recognizable Indian flavor, but if you feel a little experimental, you might want to try replacing the curry with chili powder to give it a bit of a southwestern appeal. Or if you like Cajun seasoning, try that instead of the curry (or in addition to the curry, if you really like it hot). Be bold! Play around with spices and seasonings, and you might discover you like that version of the recipe even more.

Prep time: 10 minutes; Cook time: 25 minutes (Instant Pot)
Servings: 6

1½ cup dry red lentils
1 tablespoon curry
1 large onion, chopped
½ teaspoon ginger powder
16 ounce can fire roasted tomatoes
1 head cauliflower, cut into florets

Rinse lentils, and add to an Instant Pot or other electric pressure cooker, along with the rest of the ingredients and 4 cups of water. Set timer for 25 minutes; allow pressure to come down naturally. Serve over brown rice or potato.

Option: Transfer a cup of cooked lentils to the food processor or blender, add ½ chickpeas. Blend, chill, and use as a vegetable dip.

- -

I'm Twice as Stuffed Papas Mexicanas

Most people are accustomed to that classic meal standby, rice and beans (or *arroz y frijoles*). But when you mention that you like *potatoes* and beans, they look at you like you're one bean short of a burrito. Beans and potatoes are amazing when combined, and even better when you go for the spice. If you have a bag of potatoes in your pantry and some leftover beans cooling in your fridge, you have the beginning of a beautiful food friendship. The potatoes can be cooked in advance if you are having a fiesta later.

Prep time: 15 minutes; Cook time: 90 minutes
Servings: 2 to 4

6 large russet potatoes, washed and scrubbed
1 cup or more mock refried beans
   (black or pinto)
¼ cup nutritional yeast
½ cup roasted frozen corn
2 teaspoons chili powder
2 tablespoons dried onion flakes
¼ teaspoon crushed red pepper
½ teaspoon smoked paprika
1 teaspoon lemon juice
¼ cup shredded carrots
Salsa (for garnish)

Preheat oven to 400 degrees.

Roast the potatoes in tin foil for about 1 hour. While the potatoes are cooking, mash the beans with a potato masher and add the yeast, corn, spices, and lemon juice. You don't need to fry the beans in oil to get the mouth feel of refried beans; mashing accomplishes that effect.

Remove the potatoes from oven, and take off the tin foil after the potatoes are cooled. You may refrigerate them to speed the process if you like. Once the potatoes are chilled sufficiently, cut lengthwise and scoop out the potato flesh.

Mash potato flesh and mock refried beans together, and fill potatoes. Top with shredded carrots, and then roast for an additional 20 to 25 minutes.

Top potatoes with salsa and eat!

Pass the Polenta Pizza

Ever wondered what to do with those funny-looking tubes of polenta you may have seen at your grocery? Wonder no more! Buy a couple and try this recipe. If you're a purist who wants to spend a bunch of time crafting your polenta from scratch, feel free. Meanwhile, the rest of us will be done eating while you're still boiling your corn mash. Polenta is one of those foods, like spaghetti sauce, that we prefer to buy from the store rather than make from scratch. Homemade pasta sauce is unbelievably delicious when done right; in our opinion it just takes more time than it's worth. So buy your polenta and pasta sauce without guilt. The crust for this pizza is based on corn flour and seasoned without guilt.

Prep time: 10 minutes; Cook time: 30 minutes
Servings: 2

For the crust
2 tubes polenta
½ tablespoon Italian seasoning

For the topping
6 to 8 Roma tomatoes, thinly sliced
2 garlic cloves, crushed
1 red onion, thinly sliced
1 pound crimini mushrooms, thinly sliced
1 fresh zucchini, thinly sliced
1 cup low-sodium fat-free pasta sauce
½ cup fresh arugula, snipped
½ cup fresh spinach, shipped
5 to 6 fresh basil leaves, snipped
Crushed red pepper flakes (for garnish)

Preheat oven to 425 degrees.

Squeeze the polenta into a separate medium-size bowl, and add Italian seasoning. Then add some more, if that suits you! Form the polenta mix over a pizza stone or pan.

Arrange toppings on a cookie sheet, except for the fresh greens, and lightly roast for 10 to 12 minutes. You don't want to overcook your veggies as you are going to be cooking them again with your crust.

Reduce heat to 350 degrees. Add the pasta sauce to the crust, arrange the veggies on top, and sprinkle with greens. Bake for an additional 15 minutes, or until the crust is lightly browned. Remove from the oven, and shake on crushed red pepper flakes.

- -

Inauthentic Enchilada Casserole

Inauthentic? Aren't people in the social media world constantly striving to be authentic? Well, in our experience, the people who scream authenticity are usually the biggest fakes. So why not have some fun with inauthentic enchiladas? We're using whole wheat, low-fat lavash wraps instead of "authentic" corn tortillas and cutting out cheese, meat, and oil. The lavash wraps, because they are so large, will fill your casserole pan more quickly, getting you out of the kitchen faster. Have leftovers for lunch the next day: if you bake in a toaster oven, the wraps crisp up very nicely.

> *Prep time: 15 minutes; Cook time: 30 minutes*
> 2 cups precooked pinto beans
> 1 cup precooked rice
> 1 cup fresh or frozen corn
> ½ cup shredded carrots
> 1 red and 1 green bell pepper,
>   seeded and chopped
> 2 garlic cloves, crushed
> ¼ dried onion flakes
> 2 teaspoons red pepper sauce (Tabasco)
> 2 cups homemade enchilada sauce, see page 224

1 package whole wheat lavash wraps
Chopped onions (for garnish)
Nutritional yeast (for garnish)

Preheat oven to 350 degrees.

Mash beans in a small bowl with a potato masher to a refried-bean-like texture. In a larger bowl, mix together the rice, corn, carrots, pepper, garlic, onion flakes, and red pepper sauce. Add the beans to the large bowl, and lightly mix with veggies and spices.

Pour a thin layer of the enchilada sauce into a glass 2-quart baking dish. Begin layering lavash, veggies, and sauce, until the pan is full—almost like building a lasagna.

Sprinkle chopped onions and nutritional yeast liberally on top of the casserole. Bake for 30 minutes or until the lavash crisps at the edges.

The Potato Is My Shepherd's Pie

"But what do you eat at Thanksgiving!" Not turkey! Shepherd's pie is our go-to holiday or celebration meal for a few reasons. You can make it in very large quantities ahead of time, and it's so good!

Prep time: 20 to 30 minutes; Cook time: 30 to 35 minutes
Servings: 4 to 6

10 Yukon Gold potatoes, cubed and steamed
  (no need to peel)
½ cup homemade oat milk
1 large onion, chopped
2 garlic cloves, crushed
1 sprig fresh rosemary, crushed
1 pound mushroom of choice, sliced
2 tablespoons tomato paste
2 tablespoons tamari
3 tablespoons cornstarch
4 cups cooked lentils

1 pound fresh spinach

1 pound fresh or frozen corn

Preheat oven to 400 degrees.

Mash potatoes with oat milk until fluffy and set aside. In a large wok or frying pan, sauté onions in water with garlic and rosemary until the onions are slightly soft; add mushrooms and continue to cook until the mushrooms soften as well. Add tomato paste, tamari, and cornstarch to the mixture, and cook until thickened. Stir in cooked lentils, and simmer until mixture bubbles.

Remove from the stove and set aside. Spoon the lentil mixture into a large casserole pan, and layer spinach and corn on top of the mixture. Top with mashed potatoes. Bake for 30 to 35 minutes, or until the mashed potato topping is slightly golden-brown.

SAUCES AND GRAVIES

Oh my gravy. Gravy is that delicious, gloppy, yummy topping on mashed potatoes that can suck all the health out of a perfectly good tuber. And sauces—you can quickly turn a plate of wholesome whole wheat pasta into a fatty mess. But sauces can improve the taste of a dish when prepared within our guidelines. We are only going to provide you with a few, however, because we truly want you to concentrate on keeping your meals as simple as possible. Over the next few weeks while you clear your skin, and even later, you might find that these sauces and gravies are the only ones you'll find yourself wanting or needing.

- -

KISS Enchilada Sauce

If we could find a decent enchilada sauce at the grocery, we'd recommend it. Most of the store-bought versions either contain chicken fat or oil, so we're forced back in the kitchen to make our own. We definitely believe in minimizing cooking time and maximizing your eating, working, and playing time. The joy of homemade enchiladas is worth taking the time to make this sauce, however. Feel free to double or triple the recipe and freeze the rest, so that the next time you catch an urge for enchiladas, you have a head start. We have done all that we can to speed the sauce process along. *Buena suerte!*

Prep time: 15 minutes; Cook time: 15 minutes
Servings: About 3 cups sauce

3 tablespoons chili powder

1 dried chipotle pepper, seeded, soaked, and chopped

1 teaspoon cumin

⅓ teaspoon cayenne powder

1 teaspoon garlic powder

1 teaspoon onion powder

1 to 2 tablespoons all-purpose flour or
   gluten-free flour mix

1 teaspoon arrowroot powder

2 8-ounce cans tomato paste

1½ cups low-sodium vegetable broth

Add the dried ingredients, except for the flour and arrowroot, to a blender. Grind into a fine powder. Heat the tomato paste and vegetable broth on medium high until bubbles start to form. Slowly add in the powdered spice mixture; continue to whisk lightly while the paste and broth cook. Bring to a light boil, and gradually sprinkle in the flour and arrowroot. Blend with an immersion blender while on the stove until no lumps remain. Simmer for about 10 to 12 minutes, or until the sauce is sufficiently thickened.

- -

Randa's Random Pasta Sauce

Homemade pasta sauce is definitely delicious, no question. The best sauces actually can be found simmering on a stove, literally all day. And that means you're waiting all day to eat something that is in reality a minor component of the meal. It's tasty but time waste-y. If we are going to bother making our own sauce, it has to be easy, healthy, and tasty but *not* time waste-y. Spaghetti, on the other hand, is a pretty fast food. And who doesn't love pasta? While I didn't spend the entire day simmering my sauce, my friends prefer this simple version to the store-bought alternative (which can be full of oils, meat, or dairy). I make this sauce with whatever spices are on hand. Random, in other words!

Prep time: 10 minutes; Cook time: 10 minutes
Servings: 2 to 4

2 15-ounce cans of fire-roasted tomatoes
¼ cup maple syrup
½ teaspoon dried dill
½ teaspoon ground black pepper
½ teaspoon dried thyme
1 teaspoon Italian seasoning
½ teaspoon garlic powder
Dash of salt

Heat the fire-roasted tomatoes in a saucepan on medium. Add remaining ingredients to the pan and stir until bubbles form. Blend with an immersion blender on the stove. Add pasta and eat!

- -

Cauli'Fredo Sauce

Traditional Alfredo sauce is made with heavy cream, cheese, and butter. It's like a triple bypass in a saucepan. But not to worry, you can still have a very flavorful white sauce for your pasta, without risk to your heart—or your skin.

Prep time: 10 minutes; Cook time: 5 minutes
Servings: 2 to 4

1 medium cauliflower head
3 teaspoons garlic powder
2 teaspoons onion powder
¼ cup nutritional yeast
2 tablespoons lemon juice
½ cup homemade oat milk

Steam the cauliflower until soft. Add all the ingredients to a blender, and mix on high until smooth and creamy. Reheat as necessary. Serve with pasta.

- -

Brown Is Beautiful Gravy

Gravy does *not* have to be full of fat, but it does need to be full of flavor. Arrowroot powder is your no-fat secret weapon for thickening sauces or graves. A little bit goes a long way, though.

Prep time: 10 minutes; Cook time: 10 minutes
Servings: 2 to 4

1 carton low-sodium vegetable broth
4 tablespoons all-purpose flour
2 teaspoons arrowroot powder
2 tablespoons tamari
1 tablespoon dried poultry seasoning
¼ cup dried onions

Bring the vegetable broth to a boil. Sprinkle in flour and add other ingredients. Blend with an immersion blender on the stove until the gravy is completely thickened. If you like the flavor of any one of the ingredients listed, add more. Serve over mashed potatoes, stuffing, biscuits, or basically anything you like to eat with gravy.

- -

Chi-Z Energy Sauce

Chi is the energy that animates the body—and this sauce will animate your veggies or pasta and you!

Prep time: 10 minutes; Cook time: 5 minutes
Servings: 2 to 4

1½ cups cooked white beans, drained
½ cup mashed potato (white or sweet)

½ cup homemade oat milk

½ cup nutritional yeast

2 tablespoons mellow white miso

2 tablespoons lemon juice

1 tablespoon yellow mustard

1 4-ounce jar roasted bell peppers (in water)

1 teaspoon onion powder

1 teaspoon garlic powder

Add all the ingredients to a blender along with 2 tablespoons water; blend until smooth. Warm on the stove or in a microwave. Serve over vegetables or pasta.

SNACKS AND DESSERTS

What is a snack, and what is a dessert? To us, they are both just the regular food that we eat. A snack could be portable (something you pop into your lunch bag or backpack), something you eat in between meals—but that could also be a dessert. For the purposes of the Clear Skin Diet program, we don't want you to think of snacks or desserts as some special indulgence. Perhaps they are foods on the sweeter end of the nourishment spectrum, but they are still food and nothing to feel guilty about eating—enjoy.

Some quick notes before you get into more "prepared" snack and dessert recipes. Do you really want dessert, or would your craving for something sweet be satisfied by a piece of fruit? Here are some "quickie" snack and dessert ideas.

⋄ Fruit! If you want to get a little fancy, then roll fresh or frozen strawberries or bananas in plain unsweetened cocoa powder. Most unsweetened cocoa powder contains little or no fat; chocolate only really becomes problematic when oils or other processed fats are added to it.

⋄ Frozen fruit smoothie. Add a variety of frozen fruits to a blender with water, or a plant milk of choice and ice, and blend.

⋄ Yonanas "nice" cream. Freeze bananas, process through a Yonanas machine, and add toppings. Sprinkle with cocoa powder if you need that chocolate experience. Again, this is food, but it tastes like dessert. You could eat this for breakfast.

⋄ Dates. They taste like candy wishes it could taste.

Cliff-Jumping Energy Bars

One of the foods you will typically find in vegan baking is dates, for a few reasons. Dates are naturally sweet and delicious and make a wonderful snack by themselves. Puréed, they are also an excellent replacement for oil in baking. The downside of dates is their cost; they can be quite pricey. You can easily drop ten dollars on a tiny container of dates, and you might need two or three containers for a single recipe. We decided to test baking with raisins instead, as they are significantly cheaper than dates but have a similar sticky texture and sweetness. Below is the result of our experiment. You can use the raisin paste we developed to replace dates in most recipes, and once chilled, the paste makes a nice spread on a whole wheat bagel or toast.

Prep time: 15 minutes; Cook time: 30 minutes
Servings: 6 to 8 bars

2 cups raisins (cover with water, soak overnight
  for raisin paste)
¼ cup maple syrup
1 teaspoon vanilla extract
1 teaspoon ground cinnamon
2 cups oats, divided
½ cup Grape-Nuts or Kashi 7 Whole Grain
  Nuggets cereal
½ cup fresh blueberries

This recipe works best with a food processor. Preheat oven to 425 degrees.

Drain soaked raisins; reserve water. The raisins should be plump, squishy, and rehydrated. Add soaked raisins, maple syrup, vanilla extract, and cinnamon to a food processor. Blend to a thick paste; add reserved raisin water if necessary. Remove the paste from the processor and set aside.

Add 1 cup oats and the Grape-Nuts or Kashi to the food processor (no need to clean out the paste residue), and blend to a flour-like consistency. Place mixture in a large bowl, and add the raisin paste. Stir until completely blended. Add remaining cup of oats to the mixture, and stir again. The dough should have a sticky enough texture to form into bars or balls. Add the fresh blueberries last, taking care not to squish the berries.

Form the dough into 3-inch bars; they will look very similar to the oat or energy bars you buy at the grocery store. Arrange on silicone or parchment-paper-covered cookie sheet, and bake for 30 minutes at 425 degrees. Wherever you go, these bars can go with you. Just make sure you bring enough to share.

Crazy for Cornbread

Is cornbread a snack, dessert, or a side dish? Does it matter? Just give me a piece with some homemade chili or raspberry jam.

Prep time: 10 minutes; Cook time: 20 minutes
Servings: 2 to 4

1 cup cornmeal
1 cup whole wheat pastry flour
¾ teaspoon baking soda
1 tablespoon apple cider vinegar
1 cup homemade oat milk
¼ cup applesauce
¼ cup maple syrup
½ cup fresh or frozen corn

Preheat oven to 400 degrees.

Whisk the cornmeal, flour, and baking soda together in a large bowl with a fork. Add the remaining liquid ingredients, and stir until just blended.

Pour the batter into a 9-inch glass or silicone baking dish. Bake for about 20 minutes, or until a toothpick inserted in the middle comes out clean. Double the recipe if you like, and freeze the remaining bread for a later meal.

KISS Vanilla Cake

It's your birthday! It's your birthday! Oh, my gosh, you have to have cake for your BIRTHDAY!!! Listen, guys. You can eat celebrate your birthday however you want, and it doesn't have to include cake. Sacrilege! Think about this for a sec, though. Your body shouldn't fuel itself by zip code (I'm on vacation, so I'm going to indulge in cake), the calendar (it's Harry Styles birthday, so I need to have cake), or moods (I feel happy, sad, grumpy, whatever...gimme cake). Your body works for you 24/7, and 24/7 it requires good food to keep it in good running order. OK, lecture over. Sometimes you want cake; we get it.

This is a very simple, basic, easy-to-make white cake. Save this for celebrations; this is not your daily bread. Or cake. Note: we debated over whether to provide you with frosting recipes for your cakes and decided against it. It is possible to make no-fat frostings, but they require so much sugar that we thought maybe the delight of the cake would be enough for now. While you're "on program," try "frosting" your cake with wholesome fruit spreads instead of the traditional fat-plus-sugar concoctions. You might find that you prefer fruit to frosting, anyway.

Prep time: 15 minutes; Cook time: 30 to 40 minutes
Servings: 4 to 6

2 cups all-purpose flour or gluten-free flour mix
1 teaspoon baking powder
1 teaspoon baking soda
⅓ cup unsweetened applesauce
¾ cup maple syrup
1 tablespoon vanilla extract
1 tablespoon apple cider vinegar

Preheat oven to 350 degrees.

Line an 8-inch-square cake pan with parchment paper, or use a nonstick silicone baking pan. In a medium-size bowl, sift together the flour, baking soda, and baking powder. In a smaller bowl, stir together the applesauce, maple syrup, vanilla extract, vinegar, and 1/2 cup water. Make a hole in the center of the dry ingredients, and the pour wet ingredients into the hole. Mix batter gently with cake mixer or whisk.

Add the batter to a cake pan, and bake for 30 to 40 minutes, or until a toothpick inserted into the middle comes out clean.

Option: Double the recipe for layer cake. Strawberry jam makes a delicious and surprising filling.

- -

KISS Chocolate Cake

It's your birthday! It's your birthday! Oh, my gosh, you have to have cake for your BIRTHDAY!!! Didn't we just have this discussion? Oh, but this time it's *chocolate* cake.

Prep time: 15 minutes; Cook time: 30 to 40 minutes
Servings: 4 to 6

2 cups all-purpose flour or gluten-free flour mix
1 cup no-fat unsweetened cocoa powder
1 teaspoon baking powder
1 teaspoon baking soda
⅓ cup unsweetened applesauce
¾ cup maple syrup
2 teaspoons vanilla extract
1 tablespoon apple cider vinegar

Preheat oven to 350 degrees.

Line an 8-inch-square cake pan with parchment paper or use a nonstick silicone baking pan. In a medium-size bowl, sift together the flour, cocoa powder, baking soda, and baking powder. In a smaller bowl, stir together applesauce, maple syrup, vanilla extract, vinegar, and 2/3 cup water. Make a hole in the center of the dry ingredients, and pour the wet ingredients into the hole. Mix the batter gently with a cake mixer or whisk.

Add the batter to a cake pan, and bake for 30 to 40 minutes, or until a toothpick inserted into the middle comes out clean.

Option: Double the recipe for layer cake. Raspberry jam is a particularly nice filling with chocolate.

- -

Pinch My Peach Cobbler

Here's the deal with peaches...when peaches are in season during the summer, they are so delectable, you might just gobble them up before you even make this recipe. And that's probably better for you and the peach than cooking them. Go for the fresh fruit first, is our motto. But if you want something extra special for an event or an occasion, any kind of fruit cobbler is desirable. And again, you can eat this for breakfast, because it's still "just food."

Prep time: 20 minutes; Cook time: 35 to 40 minutes
Servings: 4

5 large peaches, peeled and thinly sliced
2 tablespoons cornstarch
¼ cup frozen apple juice concentrate
1 teaspoon vanilla extract
¼ teaspoon ginger powder
¾ cup rolled old-fashioned oats
¼ cup all-purpose flour or gluten-free flour mix
1 teaspoon ground cinnamon
¼ cup maple syrup
2 tablespoons applesauce

Preheat oven to 350 degrees.

In a medium bowl, combine the peaches, cornstarch, apple juice, vanilla extract, and ginger powder. In a smaller bowl, combine the oats, flour, and cinnamon. Slowly add the maple syrup and applesauce into the oat mixture, gently mixing until thoroughly combined (this is your topping). Scoop the peach mixture into a glass or silicone 8-inch baking dish, and spread evenly throughout. Carefully top the peaches with the oat mixture.

Bake at 35 to 45 minutes. The oat mixture should be crunchy but be careful not to overcook.

- -

Mmmango Frozen Pie

Our mom created this pie for our birthday a couple of years ago because we didn't want a traditional cake. We didn't share, either! There, we admitted it. While our guests devoured vegan chocolate birthday cake, the pie was reserved for Nina and Randa.

Prep time: 15 minutes; Freeze time: 4 hours
Servings: 4 to 6

Crust
¾ cup Grape-Nuts or Kashi 7 Whole Grain Nuggets cereal
¾ cup old-fashioned rolled oats
¼ to ½ cup raisin paste (see page 229 for recipe)

Filling
2 cups frozen mangos
1 extra-ripe banana
¼ cup frozen apple juice concentrate
¼ cup maple syrup
Blueberries, strawberries, or raspberries
   (for garnish)

Process the cereal, oats, and raisin paste in a food processor until completely blended into a sticky, moldable dough. Press into a pie tin, and chill for 30 minutes in the freezer.

Add filling ingredients to a food processor or blender and mix until smooth and creamy. Pour the filling into the chilled piecrust, and allow to freeze for at least 4 hours. Decorate with fresh fruit, like blueberries, strawberries, or raspberries, before the final freeze.

- -

Black Velvet Brownies with Raspberry Sauce

We have baked these brownies for parties, but we don't tell anyone what they are made of until they are completely gone. Because, well, people get a little weirded out when they find out the chocolate brownies they just went crazy for are made with...black beans. But when you think about it, why are black beans any stranger than eating chocolate brownies made with a cup of olive oil, which takes about three pounds of olives to produce?

Prep time: 15 minutes; Cook time: 25 to 30 minutes
Servings: 6 to 8

3 cups cooked black beans, drained and rinsed
 (about two cans)
3 cups maple syrup
2 teaspoons vanilla extract
¼ cup chickpea flour beaten with ¼ cup water
2 cups fat free cocoa powder
2 cups all-purpose flour or gluten-free flour mix
2 teaspoons baking soda

Preheat oven to 350 degrees. Line a 13 x 9 x 2-inch glass baking pan with parchment paper so your brownies don't stick, or use a silicone baking pan.

Add black beans, maple syrup, vanilla extract, and chickpea flour mixture to a blender or food processor, and blend until creamy. In a separate bowl, combine the dry ingredients. Pour the dry mixture into the black bean mixture, and mix with a whisk or fork until smooth, taking care not to overmix.

Pour into a baking pan. Bake 25 to 30 minutes, or until a toothpick inserted into the middle comes out clean.

- -

Raspberry Sauce

1 bag unsweetened frozen raspberries
¼ cup maple syrup

Add ingredients to a blender along with 1/8 cup water, and blend until smooth. Serve immediately over a warm brownie.

- -

Banana Milk

OK, banana milk isn't technically a milk, but it can do a great job on your cereal. And it's sweet and contains lots of potassium and natural electrolytes, so it's one of our favorites.

>   1 banana
>   Ice (optional)
>   Dash of ground cinnamon
>   Dash of salt

Put all the ingredients along with 1 cup water and the optional ice in a blender; blend until creamy. You may want to add more or less water in order to get the consistency you like—but that's about it! Consume right away. This doesn't keep all that well in your fridge.

- -

Oat Milk

Oat milk is a healthy low-fat alternative to store-bought plant milks. Experiment with the recipe to get the consistency you prefer: more water makes it more watery, less water makes it somewhat thicker. Oat milk can be stored in the refrigerator for 4 or 5 days in mason jars or other glass containers. Be sure to stir or shake the jar before use as the milk may separate when left sitting for long periods.

>   1 cup steel-cut oats
>   1 to 2 tablespoons maple syrup or other sweetener (optional)
>   1 teaspoon vanilla extract (optional)
>   Dash of salt (optional)
>   Dash of ground cinnamon (optional)

Pour oats into a large bowl and cover with 3 cups water. Soak for about 20 minutes. Soaking overnight will produce softer oats.

Place oats and water in a blender. Start blending at low speed, gradually increasing. Blend at the highest speed for 8 to 10 seconds.

Drain oats into large bowl using a sieve, or squeeze the oats through a cheesecloth. Press the pulp with a spoon to get out as much liquid as possible, or give the cheesecloth an extra squeeze. Some people like to save the pulp for other recipes but feel free to dispose of it if you like.

Rinse the blender and pour the oat milk back in. Now you can add the rest of your optional ingredients to the oat milk and blend them together.

- -

Gluten-Free Flour Mix

Most people do not need to eat gluten-free. If you are one of those who needs to tweak your diet a bit to help heal your acne, then you can use this mix 1:1 in any recipe that calls for wheat flour.

Prep time: 5 minutes
Servings: About 10 cups

6 cups brown rice flour
2 cups potato starch
1 cup white rice flour
1 cup tapioca flour
½ cup chickpea flour

Pour ingredients into a large bowl and blend together thoroughly. Transfer to an airtight container, and shake some more. Store in a dry place; use within six months.

Acknowledgments

We don't know what our lives would have been like today had our parents not discovered John and Mary McDougall twenty-plus years ago. The incredible, lifesaving work of John and Mary has touched our family—and so many families—in countless ways. Our mom could have died a decade ago if she had not found Dr. McDougall and changed her diet. We have our mom and were able to cure our acne and conquer depression because of these two amazing people.

A huge thank you to Rip Esselstyn, who urged us to write this book and opened doors and assisted us in so many important ways in making this book happen. You rock, Rip!

We'd also like to thank the 130 Acne Intervention pilot study participants who enthusiastically participated. It's been a huge blessing to make a lot of new friends, and we're so happy and grateful they fearlessly jumped right in. Special thanks to all the people who let us use their photos in this book, in order to inspire others and illustrate the power of the Clear Skin Diet to heal acne.

We are very indebted to Steve Lawenda, MD, medical director for our Acne Intervention studies. We literally could not have done these studies without him. His enthusiasm, warmth, and expertise as a doctor and his ability to present and teach this information to participants were all key in making it a success.

We want to give a special shout-out to our team member and brother, Willie Nelson, for always being there when we need him—whether that be for taking pictures, shooting videos, hauling equipment, or just generally cheering us on. Our lifelong friend Austin Westfall and running buddy Pierre Leon seem to always show up at the right time, and our amazing team at Awesomeness TV, led by Erin Browne, has been incredibly supportive and helpful during this entire process.

We want to thank the fabulous crew at Sterling Lord Literistic: Sarah Passick, Celeste Fine, Peter Matson, and Anna Petkovich. Thank you guys so much for believing in us, for taking on the challenge to help acne sufferers around the world, and for helping bring this book into existence. We are indebted to you for all your help! Likewise, we are so grateful to the wonderful people at Hachette Books, especially our superb editor Amanda Murray. We owe a lot to Amanda for her genius suggestions and warm encouragement. Publishing maven Georgina Levitt brought incredible energy and wisdom to the promotion of the book—so many thanks due to Georgina, including bringing in PR expert Sandi Mendelson, who's opening door after door. We're likewise very appreciative of Mollie Weisenfeld, Cisca Schreefel, and Kate Mueller at Hachette.

Special thanks to our acting agents Daniel Hoff and Laura LaCombe, who continued to believe in us even when we had stopped believing in ourselves.

Thanks to the doctors, nutritionists, experts, and friends who were so supportive and contributed time and ideas for the book: Ann, Jane, Rip and Caldwell Esselstyn; Neal Barnard, MD; Chef AJ; Alona Pulde, MD; Matt Lederman, MD; Leila Masson, MD; Walter Jacobson, MD; Jeff Novick, MS, RD; Julieanna Hever, MS, RD, CPT; and Irminne Van Dyken, MD. You extraordinary people are doing so much to help humanity and the entire planet! We salute you all and are honored to call you friends.

Finally, without our parents, Jeff and Sabrina Nelson, none of this would have happened at all. We are both so appreciative that they put in hours and hours and tons of effort to help research this book, organize our Acne Intervention studies, and bring this project to fruition. We grew up watching you both follow your passion to educate others about plant-based diets, but we never really saw that as something we would end up doing ourselves. We are so happy our lives have taken this direction and that we have been able to work together with you two as a team. Thank you both for your unwavering love, support, and trips to Kauai!

—Nina and Randa

Notes

CHAPTER 1

1. Sulzberger MB, Zaidens SH. Psychogenic factors in dermatological disorders. *Med Clin North Am.* 1948;32:669–672.
2. Bhate K, Williams HC. Epidemiology of acne vulgaris. *Br J Dermatol.* 2013;168:474–485.

CHAPTER 2

1. Diaz C. *The Body Book: The Law of Hunger, the Science of Strength, and Other Ways to Love Your Amazing Body,* reprint (New York: Harper Wave, 2015).

CHAPTER 3

1. Fulton JE Jr. Effect of chocolate on acne vulgaris. *JAMA.* 1969 Dec 15;210(11):2071–2074.
2. Cordain L. Acne vulgaris: a disease of Western civilization. *Arch Dermatol.* 2002 Dec;138(12):1584–1590.
3. Rosenberg EW. Acne diet reconsidered. *Arch Dermatol.* 1981 Apr;117(4):193–195.
4. Hoehn GH. Acne and diet. *Cutis.* 1966; 2:389–394.
5. Steiner PE Necropsies on Okinawans: anatomic and pathologic observations. *Arch Pathol.* 1946;42359–42380.
6. Hoehn. Acne and diet. 389–394.
7. Mingfeng Z. Teenage acne and cancer risk in US women: a prospective cohort study. *Cancer.* 2015;121:1681–1687.
8 Sutcliffe S. Acne and risk of prostate cancer. *Int. J. Cancer.* 2007;121:2688–2692.
9. Melnik BC. Dietary intervention in acne. *Dermatoendocrinol.* 2012 Jan 1;4(1):20–32. doi: 10.4161/derm.19828.
10. Melnik BC. Are therapeutic effects of antiacne agents mediated by activation of FoxO1 and inhibition of mTORC1? *Exp Dermatol.* 2013 Jul;22(7):502–504. doi: 10.1111/exd.12172.

11.   Ibid.

12.   Cappel M. Correlation between serum levels of insulin-like growth factor 1, dehydroepiandrosterone sulfate, and dihydrotestosterone and acne lesion counts in adult women. *Arch Dermatol.* 2005 Mar;141(3):333–338.

13.   Adebamowo CA, Spiegelman D, Danby FW, Frazier AL, Willett WC, Holmes MD. High school dietary dairy intake and teenage acne. *J Am Acad Dermatol.* 2005 Feb;52(2):207–214.

14.   Farlow DW, Xu X, Veenstra TD. Quantitative measurement of endogenous estrogen metabolites, risk-factors for development of breast cancer, in commercial milk products by LC-MS/MS. *J Chromatogr. B Analyt Technol Biomed Life Sci.* 2009;877(13):1327–1334.

CHAPTER 5

1.   *A Science Odyssey: Matters of Life and Death* (PBS documentary), https://www.youtube.com/watch?v=I_xIxU7TDHE.

2.   Adams KM. Nutrition education in U.S. medical schools: latest update of a national survey. *Acad Med.* 2010 Sep; 85(9): 1537–1542.

3.   www.thepermanentejournal.org/files/Spring2013/Nutrition.pdf.

4.   Ibid.

5   Recker RR, Heaney RP. The effect of milk supplements on calcium metabolism, bone metabolism and calcium balance. *Am J Clin Nutr.* 1985 Feb;41(2):254–263.

6.   Hellerstein MK. De novo lipogenesis in humans: metabolic and regulatory aspects. *Eur J Clin Nutr.* 1999 Apr;53 Suppl 1:S53–S65; Acheson KJ, Schutz Y, Bessard T, Anantharaman K, Flatt JP, Jequier E. Glycogen storage capacity and de novo lipogenesis during massive carbohydrate overfeeding in man. *Am J Clin Nutr.* 1988 Aug;48(2):240–247; Minehira K, Bettschart V, Vidal H, Vega N, Di Vetta V, Rey V, Schneiter P, Tappy L. Effect of carbohydrate overfeeding on whole body and adipose tissue metabolism in humans. *Obes Res.* 2003 Sep;11(9):1096–1103; Dirlewanger M, di Vetta V, Guenat E, Battilana P, Seematter G, Schneiter P, Jéquier E, Tappy L. Effects of short-term carbohydrate or fat overfeeding on energy expenditure and plasma leptin concentrations in healthy female subjects. *Int J Obes Relat Metab Disord.* 2000 Nov;24(11):1413–1418; McDevitt RM, Bott SJ, Harding M, Coward WA, Bluck LJ, Prentice AM. De novo lipogenesis during controlled overfeeding with sucrose or glucose in lean and obese women. *Am J Clin Nutr.* 2001 Dec;74(6):737–746; Hellerstein MK. No common energy currency: de novo lipogenesis as the road less traveled. *Am J Clin Nutr.* 2001 Dec;74(6):707–708; Tappy L. Metabolic consequences of overfeeding in humans. *Curr Opin Clin Nutr Metab Care.* 2004 Nov;7(6):623–628.

7.   Danforth E Jr. Diet and obesity. *Am J Clin Nutr.* 1985 May;41(5 Suppl): 1132–1145.

8.   McDevitt RM, Bott SJ, Harding M, Coward WA, Bluck LJ, Prentice AM. De novo lipogenesis during controlled overfeeding with sucrose or glucose in lean and obese women. *Am J Clin Nutr.* 2001 Dec;74(6):737–746.

CHAPTER 6

1. Clark AK, Haas KN, Sivamani RK. Edible plants and their influence on the gut microbiome and acne. *Int J Mol Sci.* 2017 May 17;18(5): E1070. doi: 10.3390/ijms18051070.

CHAPTER 9

1. Golchai J. Comparison of anxiety and depression in patients with acne vulgaris and healthy individuals. *Indian J Dermatol.* 2010 Oct–Dec; 55(4): 352–354.
2. Ibid.

CHAPTER 11

1. Asawanonda P. Dark chocolate exacerbates acne. *Inter J Dermatol* 2016;55:587–591.

CHAPTER 14

1. Holt SH. A satiety index of common foods. *Eur J Clin Nutr.* 1995 Sep;49(9):675–690.
2. Mickelsen O. Effects of a high fiber bread diet on weight loss in college-age males. *Am J Clin Nutr.* 1979 Aug;32(8):1703–1709.
3. Wright N. The BROAD study: A randomized controlled trial using a whole food plant-based diet in the community for obesity, ischaemic heart disease or diabetes. *Nutr Diabetes* 2017;7: e256. doi:10.1038/nutd.2017.3 Published online 20 March 2017.

Appendix A

RECOMMENDED PRODUCTS

Please visit our website at ClearSkinDiet.com for a list of brands we have personally selected that are healthy for your skin. We plan to keep the website up to date, as products and ingredients can change.

Resources

Videos, content, skin-care product lists, and a community of people following our program can be found on our website: www.ClearSkinDiet.com.

We also have playlists of *What I Eat in a Day* videos on our YouTube channel: www.YouTube.com/NinaAndRanda.

EXPERTS WE LOVE

Neal Barnard, MD: www.PCRM.org
Ann and Caldwell Esselstyn, MD: www.DrEsselstyn.com
T. Colin Campbell, PhD: http://nutritionstudies.org/
Chef AJ: www.ChefAjWebsite.com
Jane Esselstyn, RN www.hcissc.com
Rip Esselstyn: www.Engine2Diet.com
Alan Goldhamer, DC: www.healthpromoting.com/
Julieanna Hever, MS, RD: www.PlantBasedDietitian.com
Walter Jacobson, MD: www.WalterJacobsonMD.com
Michael Klaper, MD: https://doctorklaper.com/
Matt Lederman, MD, and Alona Pulde, MD: www.WholeFoodsDiet.com
Doug Lisle, PhD: http://esteemdynamics.org/
Leila Masson, MD: www.DrLeilaMasson.com
John McDougall, MD: www.DrMcDougall.com
Jeff Novick, MS, RD: www.JeffNovick.com
Irminne Van Dyken, MD: www.OutOfTheDoldrums.com

VIDEO PROGRAMS AND EDUCATION

https://store.vegsource.com/

SOME VEGAN-ORIENTED CONTENT WE ENJOY

Our parents' website: www.VegSource.com
Our parents' YouTube channel (many expert talks): www.YouTube.com/VegSource

In addition, we recommend the following resources, listed in alphabetical order:

Tia Blanco: www.instagram.com/tiablanco

Juliet Doherty: www.instagram.com/julietdoherty

Earthy Andy: www.instagram.com/earthyandy

Ellen Fisher: www.youtube.com/user/MangoIslandMamma1

Cornelia Grismo: www.instagram.com/grimcorn/

Happy Healthy Vegan: www.youtube.com/user/HappyHealthyVegan

Jack Harries: www.youtube.com/user/JacksGap

High Carb Hannah: www.youtube.com/user/Rawkaholics

Mr. and Mrs. Vegan: www.mrmrsvegan.com/

Sophia Miacova: www.instagram.com/sophiamiacova

Kira Lynn Mukerji: www.instagram.com/kiwi.kira/

Plant-Based Athlete: www.youtube.com/user/PlantbasedAthlete

Plant-Based News: www.plantbasednews.org/

Potato Strong: www.youtube.com/user/PotatoStrong

Rawvana: www.youtube.com/user/rawvanaeng

Niomi Smart: www.youtube.com/user/niomismart

Andrew Taylor: www.spudfit.com/

Brian Turner: www.youtube.com/user/HumerusFitness

VegNews Magazine: www.VegNews.com

John Venus: www.youtube.com/user/TheQuestForFitness

FILMS/VIDEOS

Forks Over Knives: www.ForksOverKnives.com

Processed People: www.ProcessedPeople.com

What the Health: www.whatthehealthfilm.com

BOOKS

Neal Barnard, MD. *The Cheese Trap.*

Brenda Davis. *Becoming Vegan.*

Ann and Jane Esselstyn. *Prevent and Reverse Heart Disease Cookbook.*

Caldwell Esselstyn Jr., MD. *Prevent and Reverse Heart Disease.*

Rip Esselstyn. *The Engine 2 Diet* (and other books in the Engine 2 series)

Julieanna Hever, MS, RD. *The Complete Idiot's Guide to Plant-Based Nutrition.*

John McDougall, MD. *The Starch Solution* (and any other books by Dr. McDougall).

John Robbins. *The Food Revolution.*

Rich Roll. *Finding Ultra.*

Gene Stone. *Forks Over Knives: The Plant-Based Way to Health* (and other books in the Forks Over Knives series)

General Index

Recipe Index